TESTIMONIALS

"In 2003 I had the choice of spinal surgery with a 50/50 chance of success or to 'try the Pilates Studio'. I chose the latter. I was nervous of causing more damage and sceptical of achieving any improvement. Karen understood my medical condition, dealt quietly, calmly but firmly with my fears and knew when to push me to gain strength and flexibility. The result—I sleep without pain, walk the hills with no discomfort and carry my grandchildren with ease and confidence. Maintaining and improving my level of fitness has become a necessary but enjoyable way of life!"

"Joining the Pilates Studio in Taunton was the best thing I did to get rid of my back pain. Although I'd gone the usual route of physiotherapy and hydrotherapy I had reached a plateau. At Karen's Studio she used ongoing assessments to give me gentle, safe and corrective muscle-strengthening exercises. Gradually the pain became less and less and I was doing all the normal Pilates exercises. Today I'm definitely fitter and more flexible than my non-Pilates friends. And if niggles of pain return I know how to get rid of them. Karen and her trained team are really friendly, relaxed and caring of each client's needs. The sessions are always enjoyable and I look forward to each one."

"A year of attending Pilates classes has made such a difference to my hip. I was living with constant pain, but over time and with careful guidance, my core strength and flexibility has improved which supported my back and hip and relieved the pain. I didn't expect such a change as the exercises seem so subtle. The groups are small, allowing for personal attention. I cannot recommend them enough."

REHABILITATION THROUGH PILATES

REHABILITATION THROUGH PILATES
A Guide to Common Conditions

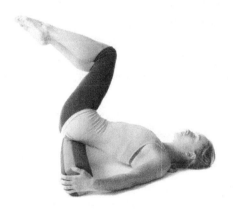

Karen Pearce and Sarah Sessa

AEON

First published in 2022 by
Aeon Books

British Library Cataloguing in Publication Data

A C.I.P. for this book is available from the British Library

ISBN-13: 978-1-80152-002-7

Typeset by Medlar Publishing Solutions Pvt Ltd, India
Printed in Great Britain

www.aeonbooks.co.uk

CONTENTS

FOREWORD   ix

INTRODUCTION   xi

PART ONE: THE BASICS

Chapter One: The basics   3

PART TWO: THE CONDITIONS

Chapter Two: Common conditions of the lumbar spine   15
Chapter Three: Common conditions of the neck   27
Chapter Four: Common conditions of the shoulder   37
Chapter Five: Common conditions of the pelvis and hip   51
Chapter Six: Common conditions of the knee and lower leg   67
Chapter Seven: Postural dysfunction   79

PART THREE: THE EXERCISES

Chapter Eight: Pelvic stability   89
Chapter Nine: The shoulder girdle   107
Chapter Ten: Spinal flexion   131
Chapter Eleven: Hip rehabilitation   145
Chapter Twelve: Spinal extension   159

Chapter Thirteen: Spinal mobilisation   169
Chapter Fourteen: Knee and lower limb   175
Chapter Fifteen: Stretches   187

RESOURCES   197

ACKOWLEDGEMENTS   199

INDEX   201

FOREWORD

For me, Pilates is not just about exercise. It is a technique, when used carefully and intelligently, can be of great benefit to society. In the present time, people lifestyle is causing more physical problems than at the time when Joseph Pilates was developing and teaching his method of exercise. The toll from bad posture and obesity is making the Pilates teacher's role more challenging and complex.

Rehabilitation Through Pilates: A Guide To Common Conditions is a life line to the majority of Pilates teachers.

Clear and concise, each condition is carefully explained, the relevant exercises clearly photographed.

This is a book for every teacher and student of Pilates and would be very useful as a homework aid for clients.

Foreward by Alan Herdman, a world renowned Pilates expert who in 1960 was invited to train in New York by teachers trained by Joseph Pilates himself. He then returned to London in 1970 to set up the UK's first Pilates studio.

INTRODUCTION

The purpose of this book and disclaimers?

We decided to write this book in order to provide a useful guide to common conditions, all of which can be helped by remedial exercise such as Pilates.

We have been specialising in rehabilitation through Pilates for many years and have gained a reputation for individualising Pilates exercise programmes to suit different issues. We have many thankful clients who attend the studios regularly and are now able to continue with their hobbies and activities without the pain they had previously been suffering.

In this book we have not only set out remedial exercises for the common conditions but also provided a detailed anatomy and pathology breakdown for each. We feel it is necessary for an exercise practitioner to understand the anatomy behind the condition to properly attempt to remedy it.

The principles and fundamentals of Pilates should already be understood before attempting the exercises in this book as it is aimed at the more experienced instructor or client. Although most of the conditions are set out clearly with contraindications and suggested exercises, it is always necessary to get a referral from a professional medical practitioner before undertaking any exercise.

The exercises suggested in this book are relevant to each condition but are not complete Pilates exercise programmes, therefore they should be included in a more general programme to encompass an overall individualised approach to Pilates exercise.

This book is written for Pilates instructors and also clients who are keen to know more about their condition. This is why we only offer brief descriptions of non-Pilates management so that the reader can become a little familiar with other procedures that might be in place. Information about non-Pilates management in this book is based on clinical practice and the most recent National Institute for Health and Care Excellence (NICE) guidelines as available at the time of writing this book (2020). However, it is important to recognise that this is a Pilates book that does not aim to offer physiotherapists (or similar professionals) a therapeutic treatment textbook. Having said that, therapists may find this book of interest from a Pilates perspective.

Within the text we often words about following the advice and guidance of the physiotherapists, but we are aware that clients may have seen alternative disciplines such as an osteopath or sports therapist so in that case we advise you to follow the guidance of those professionals.

PART ONE

THE BASICS

CHAPTER ONE

The basics

Balance of body: the Pilates method

"A balance of body and mind"

Joseph Pilates was born in 1883 in Germany: he was a sickly child and grew up determined to improve his physical ability. He came to England just before the First World War and because of his nationality he was interned at a hospital where he was required to offer rehabilitation to war veterans. His famous Universal Reformer machine was originally invented after attaching springs to hospital beds to allow those confined to bed to exercise. After the war Pilates returned to Germany and soon after that moved to New York where he devised an exercise regime called Contrology which he developed from watching animals stretch, practising self-defence, acrobatics, boxing, and eventually working with leading ballet dancers of the time. Contrology was based on the principles of muscle balance, core strength, and agility—an exercise system that required thought too. Joseph Pilates felt strongly that his exercise was to be used in everyday life—as a way of life!

The Pilates that is practised today has the advantage of being used and improved by physiotherapists and other medical professionals, and as we gain greater knowledge of the human body these techniques are improved. However, the fundamentals of Joseph Pilates's exercise regime remain the same: "a balance of body and mind" and his six principles.

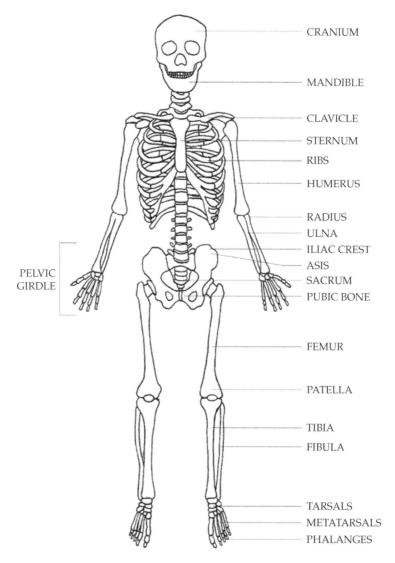

Figure 1. Front of skeleton.

The six principles of Pilates

Breath

A good breathing pattern will stop your breath becoming tense and shallow which will cause even simple things such as climbing stairs to become difficult. Learning to control your breathing will allow movements to become more natural and relaxed.

With Pilates exercises we mainly use lateral breathing which is a breath into the sides of the ribcage as opposed to expanding the abdomen (or pushing out the tummy);

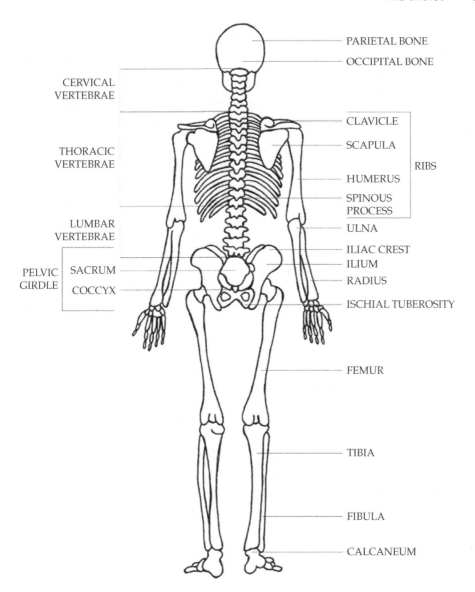

Figure 2. Back of skeleton.

this enables the deep abdominal muscles to be engaged on both inhalation and exhalation which helps to stabilise the pelvic girdle (strengthen the core muscles).

Concentration

Having to isolate certain muscles also focuses the mind. Thinking about the breathing pattern, which muscles are being activated, and the correct alignment of the body will improve concentration. As you become more proficient at the exercises you will begin to realise how the mind can control our movements—it's just a matter of connecting mind to body.

Centre

Strength is coming from a central point of your body which is your core. To feel that your body is centred means that the muscles are balanced and the core muscles are strong. This allows you to maintain a correct posture and undertake everyday activities without causing injury to vulnerable places such as the spine. Practising Pilates will improve the way you stand and eliminate muscular pain caused by bad posture.

Control

The Pilates method uses the mind and body to obtain complete control of the exercises. This will lead to improving strength, flexibility, co-ordination and balance.

Precision

Pilates exercises are mainly small, very subtle movements; precision is more important than repetition. Total concentration and focus is necessary to control pace, breath, alignment, posture, and use of the core.

Flow

If all the other principles are adhered to Pilates exercises should flow from one to another with controlled yet flowing movements.

Pilates fundamentals

Alignment

Correct alignment, both static and dynamic is necessary throughout a Pilates practice to achieve the desired results in each and every part of the exercises.

Breathing

Lateral or thoracic breathing is taught for most Pilates exercises in order to maintain core stability throughout the movements.

Centring

Movements should be controlled from the centre or core to properly execute exercises for both mobility and stability.

Muscle balance

In order to achieve an optimum posture that is as close to "ideal" as possible, the muscles need to be activated properly and efficiently so as to avoid pain and injury: this is what we think of as muscle balance.

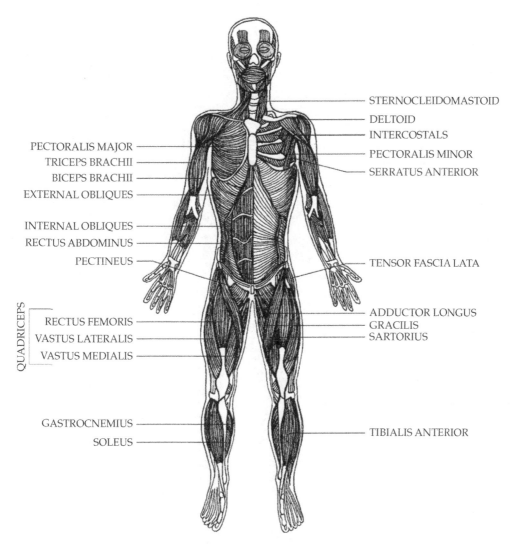

Figure 3. Muscles (front).

Pilates exercises are mainly small, very subtle movements and precision is more important than repetition. We can get into bad postural habits and allow some muscles to become over strong and tight, and others weak and underused.

Acquiring an understanding of which muscles should be working and isolating these muscles will correct these issues. Although it seems difficult at first this ability to isolate muscles improves with practice and once mastered can be taken into every aspect of daily life.

When practising the Pilates exercises regularly you will gradually improve to achieve the desired amount of control. The muscles will become more balanced so that the stronger ones don't dominate, and you will start to feel in control of your

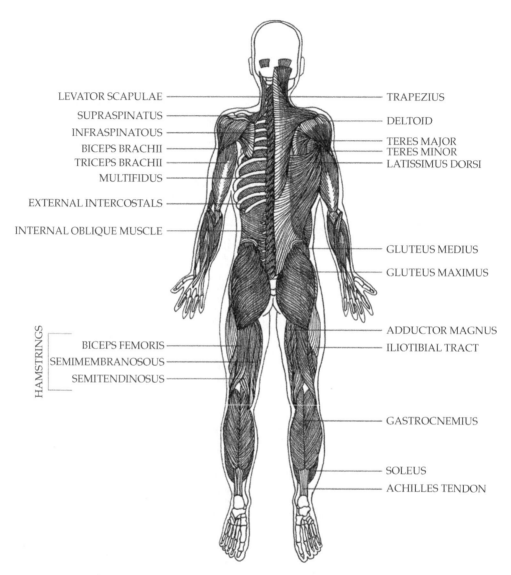

Figure 4. Muscles (back).

movements. Eventually the programme of exercises will become more natural and require less of a conscious effort.

As we get older our joints start to stiffen, we move less and so lose flexibility. This is unnecessary; if we keep our joints moving and muscles stretched, we can continue to stay flexible, maintain an upright posture, and retain agility into old age. This is all the more achievable if a Pilates routine is practised regularly and becomes a way of life.

From our study of anatomy we learn that muscles have different fibre types depending on their function: local stabiliser muscles are designed for endurance and lie close to the joint providing stability and support. Transversus abdominus and multifidus are examples of local stabilisers and work together to maintain correct posture.

Sometimes these muscles don't work correctly due to a variety of factors: perhaps a client has arthritis that causes pain, thus altering joint position or weight-bearing, or perhaps they have a neurological condition that affects muscle control. Either of these scenarios will cause muscle imbalance where the local stabilisers no longer offer the stability that they should and altered posture results. Global (or secondary) stabilisers are not as deep as the local stabiliser muscles and their function is to help with motor control turning "on and off" depending on the movement that is taking place rather than the sustained, low-level contraction of the local stabilisers. Examples are gluteus maximus and the external obliques. If these muscles don't produce enough force, they can't provide adequate control and become shaky. Finally, global mobilisers are muscles that work under increased load and produce high power but minimal endurance. They are positioned superficially and can quickly build up tension; however, they can become tight when overused or used incorrectly. Examples of global mobilisers are the hamstrings and the rectus abdominus. Several muscles can have two roles, working as a global stabiliser or mobiliser depending on the situation.

Posture

Posture is the position in which we hold our body when up against gravity and can be considered in standing, sitting, or lying. It is normal to have curves throughout the spine: the cervical and lumbar areas have a natural lordosis, and the thoracic, sacral, and coccygeal areas have a natural kyphosis. The problems arise when these curves become either increased or decreased, putting stress and pressure on surrounding anatomical structures. It isn't just incorrect positions of the spine that can lead to problems: any joint malalignment or sub-optimal muscle length or function will also contribute.

Posture is considered to be "good" when the bones and joints are kept in optimal alignment and there is as little stress as possible on supporting muscles and ligaments. When standing in the anatomical position, that is, standing with the feet hip-width apart and the arms by the side with the palms facing forwards, an ideal posture would be as follows: the feet are almost parallel with only a slight turn out; the weight of the body is evenly distributed through the right and left; weight is neither too far forwards on the balls of the feet or too far back on the heels; the kneecaps face forwards and during a small knee bend each kneecap is directed over the second toe; the pelvis is in a neutral position with the pubic symphysis in the same plane as the anterior superior iliac spines: the natural curves of the spine are maintained throughout; the ribs don't flare and there is a gentle connection between the bottom of the sternum and the pubic symphysis; the collar bones are wide and open; the shoulders are relaxed and not hunched up or rounded; the shoulder blades are equidistant from the vertebral column and in contact with the thorax, gently drawing down the back; lastly the head sits centrally and the chin is not poking forwards. However, it is very unusual to find someone that has this ideal posture, and our aim is not to try to achieve this as that would be unrealistic, rather it is to try to achieve the best posture possible for each individual.

In very simplistic terms there are four main posture types that can lead to problems: lordotic, flat back, kyphotic, and sway back, as shown in Figure 5.

As we will go on to discover later in the "Postural dysfunction" chapter, there are many factors that contribute to posture and individuals very rarely fit into one simple type. However, becoming familiar with these four basic posture types is a good place to start.

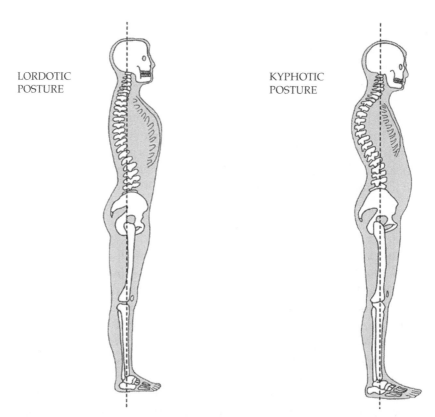

LORDOTIC
POSTURE

KYPHOTIC
POSTURE

Figure 5a. Hyper-lordosis.

Figure 5b. Hyper-kyphosis.

Can be seen in dancers, pregnancy, obesity, gymnasts. The natural lordosis is exaggerated so low back extensors such as erector spinae are tight; the pelvis is tilted anteriorly; the rectus abdominus and external obliques are lengthened; the hamstrings can be tight in the knee region but lengthened in the hip region; hip joints are in flexion with tight hip flexors; hip adductors can be tight.	Can be seen in office workers, increased computer or mobile phone use/texting, people who are tall. The natural kyphosis of the thoracic spine is exaggerated; the chin pokes forward with the neck in hyperextension so that the neck extensors are short and tight; the deep neck flexors are long and weak; the shoulders are rounded forwards with tight pectorals; shoulder blades are abducted with weak and lengthened scapula stabilising muscles.

SWAY BACK
POSTURE

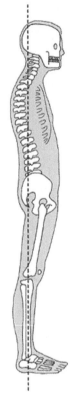

FLAT-BACK
POSTURE

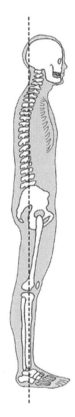

Figure 5c. Sway back.

Figure 5d. Flat back.

This posture might be seen in teen-agers or people that stand for a long time and sway their pelvis forwards appearing to rest on their hip liga-ments. The lumbar spine is flat; the pelvis is posteriorly tilted with long, weak hip flexors; the oblique abdomi-nals are shortened; knees are hyper-extended but the hamstrings may actually be shortened and tight in the hip region; intercostals are tight.

There is lack of mobility in the lumbar spine and is seen in those that do a lot of abdominal crunches or sports such as boxing. The rectus abdominus and hamstrings are tight; hip flexors are long and weak; posterior pelvic tilt with slight lengthening of the erector spinae.

PART TWO

THE CONDITIONS

CHAPTER TWO

Common conditions of the lumbar spine

Relevant anatomy and movement
    Common conditions:

1. Non-specific low back pain
2. Disc prolapse
3. Facet joint syndrome
4. Degenerative joint disease: osteoarthritis and spondylosis
5. Spondylolysis and spondylolisthesis
6. Stenosis

Anatomy of the lumbar spine

The vertebral column is made up of thirty-three vertebrae that link together through intervertebral joints: the synovial articular facet joints and the fibrocartilaginous disc joints. There are seven cervical vertebrae, twelve thoracic vertebrae, five lumbar vertebrae, five fused sacral vertebrae and three to four coccygeal vertebrae that are all or partially fused. Between each vertebra and the one below there are two facet joints and one fibrocartilaginous joint which is where we find the intervertebral disc. As the bones link together a protective canal is formed, from the occiput of the skull all the way down to the last lumbar vertebrae (L5) that offers protection to the delicate spinal cord. At each vertebral level spinal nerves exit the canal via the intervertebral foramen.

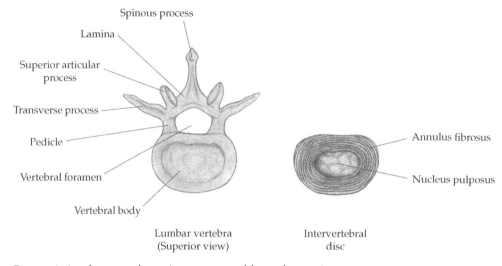

Lumbar vertebra
(Superior view)

Intervertebral
disc

Figure 6. Lumbar vertebrae (posterior and lateral views).

   The lumbar spine consists of five large and strong vertebrae (L1–L5) that are designed to support the weight of the upper body. Each vertebra has one large quadrilateral spinous process and two relatively long transverse processes that provide sturdy attachment for the powerful muscles of the lower back. The fifth lumbar vertebra (L5) is the largest of the five and has the most substantial transverse processes. In between the vertebrae there is an intervertebral disc which is made up of an outer fibrocartilaginous ring that surrounds a central gel-like inner structure called the nucleus pulposus. The purpose of the disc is to provide shock absorption.

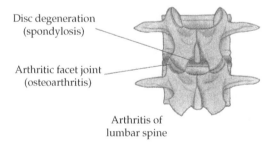

Arthritis of
lumbar spine

Figure 7. Lumbar vertebra (superior view) and intervertebral disc.

Movement

The spine when moving as a whole has a large range of movement (ROM) which is evident in the way we can bend to pick something up from the floor (flexion), turn to reach for something from behind (rotation), or stretch up high (extension). This gross movement is the sum of small, segmental movements occurring at each vertebral level. At the lumbar spine deep muscles posteriorly such as multifidus and rotatores are close to the intervertebral joints and provide stability (as well as providing segmental extension and rotation respectively) and anteriorly our main core stability muscle is transversus abdominus. As muscles become more superficial, they act as mobilisers, contributing to larger movements of the spine.

Flexion: Rectus abdominus and psoas major.

Extension: Erector spinae, quadratus lumborum also assists.

Side flexion: External and internal obliques of the same side, quadratus lumborum.

Rotation: Gross rotation of the lower half of the spine, for example rotation to the left, is caused by the left internal oblique and right external oblique. This is limited at the lumbar spine due to inward-facing facets.

Conditions of the lumbar spine

For the purpose of this book we mention three main causes of low back pain (LBP):

- **Systemic** in origin, for example related to malignancy or sepsis (infection). This is not discussed here as we are very unlikely to come across these cases in our Pilates practice as this will have been picked up by a medical professional. As with all conditions, if in any doubt refer the client back to their doctor.
- **Non-specific LBP.**
- **Structural** in nature, for example facet joint arthritis, prolapsed intervertebral disc (PID), inflammatory processes or spondylolisthesis.

Various tissues may be the origin of LBP, for example torn or strained muscle fibres or ligaments; damage to the discs; inflammation or strain of the facet joints; inflammation, compressions or entrapment of the nerves, or injuries such as subluxation or fractures of the vertebrae.

1. Non-specific low back pain (NSLBP)

NSLBP is thought to affect one third of the population each year. In 2016 the National Institute for Health and Care Excellence (NICE) updated its guidelines to place much more emphasis on suitable exercise programmes such as "biomechanical, aerobic, mind-body or a combination of approaches".

People who are considered to have NSLBP are often recommended to try Pilates after assessment and treatment by their doctor and physiotherapist (or similar healthcare professional). In these cases, back pain is often due to poor posture or poor lifting technique associated with everyday life or occupation. Muscle strain leads to incorrect muscle activity and muscle imbalance which can lead to poor joint alignment and pain arising from the intervertebral discs, facet joints, and other local structures. Usually, any inflammation will resolve and exercises to correct posture and stability are advised.

Presentation: The client can present with stiffness, pain, muscle tension, and spasm in the lumbar region, sometimes referring into the lower limbs.

Management: Pain relief, exercise, physiotherapy, lifestyle advice.

| Pilates programme for **lower back pain** | Initially strengthen the core muscles to activate transversus abdominis and stabilise the pelvis, also work to lengthen the lumbar extensors and hip flexors in order to address muscle imbalance that will in turn improve and maintain joint alignment. Eventually progress to a more general programme but focus on abdominal strength and lumbar spinal flexion. |
| Contraindications/ cautions | Avoid spinal extension if posture is lordotic and spinal extensors are tight as extension may contribute to further tightness and exacerbate symptoms. |

Initial exercises recommended	Chapter	Exercise no.	Page no.
• Breathing and static abs (transversus activation)	8	1	91
• Leg slides	8	4	93
• Small tilts	10	35	131
• Small tilts on soft ball	10	36	132
• Abdominal exercise with gym ball/roller	8	8	95
• Chest lifts	10	39	134
• Lumbar circles	13	72	170
• Lumbar stretch	15	96	196
• Iliopsoas stretch	15	86, 87	188, 189

Progression			
• Pelvic tilts seated on reformer	10	38	133
• Oblique chest lifts	10	40	135
• Curl down on trapeze	10	42	136
• Curl down (half) with TheraBand	10	41	136
• Cat on reformer	10	44	139
• Tippy toes on soft ball	8	14	105
• Psoas stretch and lumbar stretch (on soft ball)	15	86	188
• Lumbar stretch seated on reformer	10	46	142
• Thread the needle (flexion part only if tightness in spinal extensors)	13	71	169
• Buttock stretch	15	90	191

2. Prolapsed intervertebral disc (PID), also known as a slipped disc, or herniated disc Although low back pain is very common, only a few cases are thought to be due to a disc prolapse. PID occurs most frequently in the lumbar spine with highest incidence at L4–5 or L5–S1 (sacral vertebra one). The cause of a prolapsed disc is unclear but typically, there is a weakness or degeneration of the outer layer of the disc which causes the nucleus pulposus to herniate and press on nearby structures including the nerve roots. This can happen as a consequence of too much pressure on the weakened disc

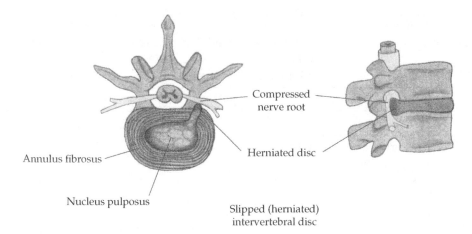

Compressed nerve root

Herniated disc

Annulus fibrosus

Nucleus pulposus

Slipped (herniated)
intervertebral disc

Figure 8. Prolapsed intervertebral disc.

during activities that require awkward bending or lifting, or even a job that requires prolonged sitting. Lifestyle factors such as smoking and obesity may contribute.

Presentation: PID is more commonly seen in male clients and people between the ages of thirty and fifty, and they may or may not be able to recall a specific incident that led to the onset of pain. Pain is generally made worse with flexion activities such as sitting and bending and there may be muscle spasm, radiculopathy (pain along the path of a nerve) as in sciatica, or leg pain in the sciatic nerve root distribution. There may be other nerve root signs such as weakness or altered sensation in the buttock, hamstring, calf, and foot. Pain is relieved by changing position or lying down, and coughing or sneezing can exacerbate the pain. Very rarely cauda equina syndrome can occur which is a medical emergency where the nerve roots coming out of the base of the spine are compressed, leading to bladder and bowel problems, numbness in the saddle area, or weakness in one or both legs. The client must see a doctor immediately as surgery might be needed to avoid permanent damage.

Management: Most cases of PID will resolve spontaneously within a few weeks. They may benefit from pain relief, physiotherapy, and encouragement to keep moving and exercise. Investigations such as X-rays and scans are not routinely used unless symptoms persist. The scans will then be useful to help establish the size and position of the disc prolapse and whether surgery is indicated.

Pilates programme for **prolapsed intervertebral disc**	Initially avoid spinal flexion and work to stabilise the pelvis by strengthening the core and local stability muscles particularly transversus abdominis and multifidus. Once strength is gained and any muscle imbalance of the trunk and pelvis is addressed start to add gentle flexion to mobilise the spine. Eventually work towards a more general programme keeping focus on the co-contraction of abdominals and back extensors.

(Continued)

Contraindications/ cautions	Avoid spinal flexion whilst it exacerbates back or leg pain but don't avoid indefinitely. Start slowly with flexion exercises (pelvic tilts etc.) only once pain is gone or on the advice of a physiotherapist.

Exercises recommended	Chapter	Exercise no.	Page no.
• Static abs work–transversus and pelvic floor activation in neutral	8	1, 2	91
• Leg slides	8	4	93
• Knee lifts	8	7	94
• Abdominal exercise with gym ball/roller	8	8	95
• Bridge	8	11	102
• Prone gluteal squeeze	11	55	152
• Prone hamstring curls	11	56	152
• Swimming prep	12	62	159
• Dart	12	63	160
• Prancers	8	10	102

Progression			
• Small pelvic tilts	10	35	131
• Chest lifts	10	39	134
• Mini curl up on trapeze	10	45	140
• Tippy toes on soft ball	8	14	105
• Arrow	12	65	161
• Cobra	12	66	162
• Swan prep on reformer	12	67	163
• Swan on combo chair	12	68	165
• Leg work on reformer	8	9a, 9b, 9c	96, 98, 99
• Prancers	8	10	102
• Superman	12	69	166
• Superman on reformer	12	70	167
• Kneeling plank on reformer	8	13	104

3. Facet joint syndrome

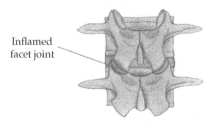

Inflamed
facet joint

Figure 9. Facet joint syndrome.

The small, synovial facet joints of the lumbar spine can become irritated and inflamed due to poor posture (mostly commonly with increased lordosis), osteoarthritis, or less likely from trauma.

Presentation: Generally, pain occurs during extension or side flexion to the affected side. Pain and stiffness can become constant with time.

Management: Pain relief, physiotherapy

Pilates Programme for **facet joint** syndrome:	Work to open up the facet joints through gentle flexion and soft ball exercises. Progress to strengthening abdominals and lengthening hip flexors and lumbar extensor muscles to improve posture.
Contraindications/ cautions	Avoid spinal extension.

Exercises recommended	Chapter	Exercise no.	Page no.
• Pelvic tilts on soft ball	10	36	132
• Pelvic tilts	10	35	131
• Butterfly on soft ball	8	15	106
• SI joint rolling and walking on roller (across sacrum)	15	91	162
• Cat (no extension)	10	43	138
• Thread the needle (flexion part only)	13	71	169
• Lumbar circles	13	72	170
• Lumbar stretch	15	96	196

Progression			
• Seated pelvic tilts on Reformer	10	38	133
• Cat on reformer	10	44	139
• Chest lifts	10	39	134
• Tippy toes on soft ball	8	14	105
• Curl down with TheraBand	10	41	136
• Curl down on trapeze	10	42	136
• Leg work on reformer	8	9a, 9b	96, 98
• Iliopsoas stretches	15	86–89	188–190

4. Degenerative joint disease: osteoarthritis and spondylosis

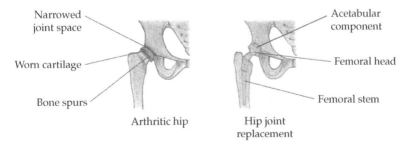

Figure 10. Arthritis of the lumbar spine.

Osteoarthritis and spondylosis are both considered as degenerative joint diseases that may occur independently or in association with each other. Either way it is important to note the difference between the two types: osteoarthritis occurs at the synovial facet joints whereas spondylosis is degeneration that occurs around the cartilaginous (i.e. non-synovial) intervertebral discs. With facet joint arthritis osteophytes can form that compress on the nerve roots or more centrally leading to spinal stenosis. With spondylosis there is degeneration around the discs which may consist of osteophyte formation at the vertebral bodies, narrowed disc spaces, sclerotic vertebral bodies and decreased water content of the disc with annular tears.

Presentation: Clients with degenerative changes describe symptoms such as pain, aching, stiffness, and loss of movement. Facet joint arthritis can present as facet joint syndrome.

Pilates programme for **degenerative joint disease**: osteoarthritis and spondylosis	If facet joint syndrome presents, then aim to open up joints as described previously. In addition, aim to mobilise the lumbar region, strengthen core muscles, and lengthen any tight muscles.
Contraindications/ cautions	Avoid spinal extension if facet joint syndrome symptoms are evident.

Exercises recommended	*Chapter*	*Exercise no.*	*Page no.*
• Static abs (transversus and pelvic floor activation)	8	1, 2	91
• Pelvic tilts	10	35	131
• Small pelvic tilts on soft ball	10	36	132
• Leg slides	8	4	93
• Knee lifts	8	7	94
• Abdominal exercise with gym ball/roller with modification to slight posterior tilt	8	8	95
• Chest lifts	10	39	134
• Curl down (half) with TheraBand	10	41	136
• Cat (no extension)	10	43	138
• Lumbar stretch	15	96	196
• Lumbar circles	13	72	170
Progression			
• Butterfly on soft ball	8	15	106
• Bug exercise	8	5	93
• Oblique chest lifts	10	40	135
• Leg work on reformer	8	9a, 9b	96, 98
• Pelvic curls seated on reformer	10	38	133
• Lumbar stretch seated on reformer	10	46	142
• Lumbar stretch seated on a gym ball	10	47	142

5. Spondylolysis and spondylolisthesis

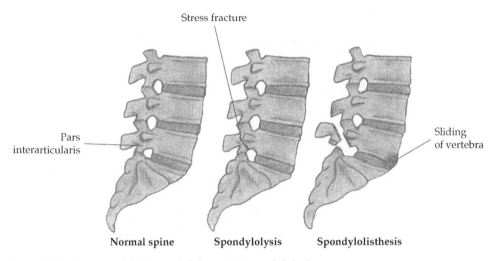

Figure 11. a) Normal b) Spondylolysis c) Spondylolisthesis.

Spondylolysis is a condition where there is a defect in the pars interarticularis (PI) which is part of the facet joint structure. It is commonly found in the sporting (mostly adolescent) population, particularly where there is repetitive loading into rotation and extension, for example, cricketers, athletes and gymnasts. Associated micro-trauma and stress fractures of the PI can occur most commonly at the level of L5. Twenty-five per cent of patients present with symptoms such as pain and stiffness, whilst others remain asymptomatic. If the vertebra is affected bilaterally then spondylolysis can progress to spondylolisthesis. Spondylolisthesis means slipping of the vertebra, more specifically the vertebra above slips forward on the vertebra below. This can occur for a number or reasons:

- Congenital deficiency of the lumbo-sacral facets (rare)
- Progression of spondylolysis (most common cause)
- Degeneration due to mechanical wear of the posterior facet joints, mostly seen in women over the age of fifty-five
- Trauma
- Pathology (e.g. a tumour or osteoporosis).

Presentation: Spondylolysis can be asymptomatic, or clients may describe a non-traumatic, slow onset with localised LBP that increases with activity, especially lumbar extension movements. With spondylolisthesis the spine might be tender at the midline and the clinician may feel a "step" at the affected level. Pain increases with lumbar spine extension, but flexion is not usually painful. There may be increased lordosis but usually no nerve root pain unless there is root compression at the site of the lesion. If the spondylolisthesis is sport-related the presentation will be that of spondylosis.

Management: Activity restriction, rest, and physiotherapy are advised with possible surgery if there is no improvement after substantial conservative (non-surgical) management.

Depending on our place of work we are most likely to come across those with a degenerative spondylolisthesis. For the sport-related spondylolysis or spondylolisthesis be guided by the client's physiotherapist as to when they can start a Pilates programme. The physiotherapist may recommend specific exercises especially if they have to rehabilitate back to a particular sport.

Pilates programme for **spondylolysis and spondylolisthesis**	Work to stabilise the pelvis by strengthening core muscles particularly transversus abdominis and multifidus but avoid spinal extension. Progress to more abdominal strengthening and isometric work such as bridge and planks when (if) able.
Contraindications/ cautions	Avoid spinal extension.

Exercises recommended	*Chapter*	*Exercise no.*	*Page no.*
• Small tilts	10	35	131
• Small tilts on soft ball	10	36	132
• Leg slides	8	4	93
• Knee lifts	8	7	94
• Abdominal exercise with gym ball/roller with modification to slight posterior tilt	8	8	95
• Leg work on reformer	8	9a, 9b, 9c	96, 98, 99
• Curl down (half) with TheraBand	10	41	136
• Chest lifts	10	39	134
• Cat (no extension)	10	43	138
• Cat on reformer	10	44	139
• Lumbar stretch	15	96	196
• Lumbar stretch seated on reformer	10	46	142
Progression			
• Large pelvic tilts	10	37	132
• Mini curl up on trapeze	10	45	140
• Oblique sit ups	10	40	135
• Curl down on trapeze	10	42	136
• Bridge	8	11	102
• Bridge on trapeze	8	12	103
• Tippy toes on soft ball	8	14	105
• Kneeling plank on reformer	8	13	104

6. Spinal stenosis

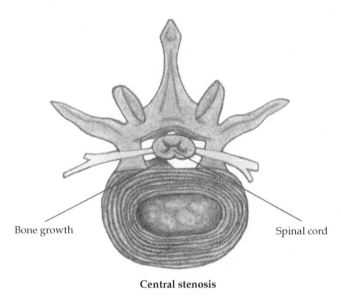

Central stenosis

Figure 12. Spinal stenosis.

This is narrowing of the vertebral foramen or canal which can be congenital (born with) or acquired. It can occur in the cervical spine but is more common in the lumbar region.

Examples of acquired causes are:

- Due to degeneration and osteophytes that encroach into the canal
- Posterior vertebral slipping that occurs in spondylolisthesis
- PID that herniates directly posteriorly.

As the space narrows there is compression of the spinal cord and nerve roots.

Presentation: Back pain, buttock pain, tingling, cramping leg pain and pain on standing and walking or radiculopathy. Walking and standing tend to make the symptoms worse as the vertebral canal narrows in these extension activities. Sitting down can help to relieve symptoms as the vertebral canal widens.

Management: Conservative management such as exercise may be sufficient but if symptoms persist spinal injections may be considered to alleviate pain, or decompression surgery to relieve pressure on the canal structures.

Flexion exercises will help to open up the canal, but extension will exacerbate symptoms as the canal size reduces. We want to work on the core and posture to stabilise the area in order to try to maintain a more "open" vertebral canal.

| Pilates programme for **spinal stenosis** | Initially use gentle spinal flexion exercises. Work on stabilising the pelvis and strengthening the core to improve posture and restrict tightening of the lumbar spine. Be careful of introducing too many spinal extension exercises even when stronger. |
| Contraindications/ cautions | Avoid spinal extension. |

Exercises recommended	Chapter	Exercise no.	Page no.
• All pelvic stabilisation exercises (except bridge)	8	1–10	91–102
• Pelvic tilts	10	35	131
• Small pelvic tilts on soft ball	10	36	132
• Abdominal exercise with gym ball/roller with modification to slight posterior tilt	8	8	95
• Curl down (half) with TheraBand	10	41	136
• Tippy toes on soft ball	8	14	105
• Lumbar and psoas stretch on soft ball	15	88	190
• Cat (no extension)	10	43	138
• Cat on reformer	10	44	139
• Lumbar stretch	15	96	196
Progression			
• Larger pelvic tilts	10	37	132
• Curl down on trapeze	10	42	136
• Chest lifts	10	39	134
• Oblique sit-ups	10	40	135
• Thread the needle (flexion part only)	13	71	169

CHAPTER THREE

Common conditions of the neck

Relevant anatomy and movement
   Common conditions of the neck

1. Degenerative joint disease: osteoarthritis and spondylosis
2. Whiplash
3. Disc prolapse
4. Torticollis
5. Cervicogenic headaches

Anatomical structures of the cervical spine

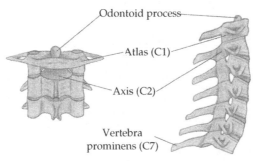

Cervical vertebrae
(Posterior view)

Cervical vertebrae
(Right lateral view)

Figure 13. Cervical vertebrae (posterior and lateral views).

The seven cervical vertebrae are small and light in relation the thoracic and lumbar and are designed for mobility. The first two vertebrae, named the atlas and axis and C7 differ in design to vertebrae C3–C6. C1 (the atlas) meets with the occiput of the skull forming the atlanto-occiput joint; there is no body, but instead a large vertebral foramen (hole) which allows the passage of the spinal cord as it exits skull via the foramen magnum.

The transverse processes are large which helps with rotation of the head. There is a facet on the anterior arch of C1 that provides a surface for the odontoid peg of the axis to move on, allowing rotation of the head on the neck.

C2 (the axis) has a very small body, small bifid spinous process and its characteristic odontoid peg which represents the atlas vertebral body and allows for rotation as described above. C3 to C6 are similar to each other in design with a vertebral body, bifid spinous process, right and left transverse process, and a relatively large vertebral canal. C7 (vertebra prominens) has a long, non-bifid spinous process which offers a useful bony landmark. The cervical vertebrae have a transverse foramen which houses the vertebral arteries, except C7 where the foramen may be basic or absent with no vertebral vessels passing through.

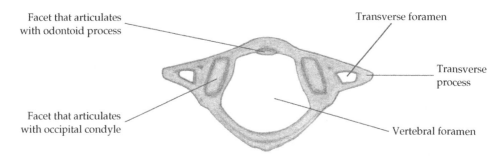

Figure 14. Atlas (superior view).

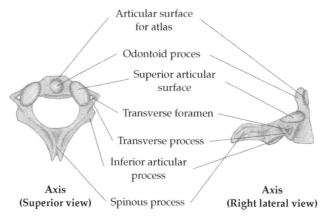

Figure 15. Axis (superior and lateral views).

Movements and muscles of the cervical spine and head

Flexion: Longus capitis, rectus capitis anterior, sternocleidomastoid (SCM), longus colli, scalenes

Extension: Semispinalis capitis, longissimus capitis, splenius capitis, spinalis capitis, semispinalis cervicis

Side flexion: Rectus capitis lateralis, SCM, scalenes

Rotation: SCM (to opposite side), longissimus capitis, longissimus cervicis, semispinalis cervicis

As for the lumbar spine the deep multifidus and rotatores will help stabilise and aid with extension and rotation at a segmental level.

Common conditions of the neck

Research shows that neck pain is very common. Exact figures are hard to ascertain due to varied data, but you will certainly come across many clients on a weekly, if not daily basis who are complaining of neck discomfort. A substantial number of these clients will experience a recurrence of symptoms but we, as instructors, can really help to prevent this by providing suitable exercise programmes and advice. Most neck pain is "non-specific" where there is pain and discomfort in the neck and possibly the shoulder girdle with or without pain referred to the arms. Symptoms vary with activity and over time. In most cases, the exact cause of neck pain is hard to identify but fortunately serious causes are rare with the most likely cause being mild strain to local structures such as the small joints and ligaments. Prolapsed discs and nerve damage, despite being more serious than in the lumbar spine, are less common.

For simplicity we will consider neck pain as three groups, as we did for the lumbar spine:

- **Systemic** in origin, for example malignancy or sepsis. This is not in our remit to manage through Pilates.
- **Structural** in nature, such as arthritis, prolapsed-intervertebral disc (PID), inflammatory processes, stenosis, torticollis or "wry neck", or injuries such as whiplash.
- **Non-specific pain** due to poor posture, neck strain, sport, occupation, sedentary lifestyle, and stress. This will be covered in the upper crossed syndrome of Chapter Seven.

1. Degenerative joint disease: osteoarthritis and spondylosis
As for the lumbar spine, osteoarthritis and spondylosis are both considered as degenerative joint disease and can occur together. Osteoarthritis occurs at the synovial facet joints whereas spondylosis is degeneration that occurs around the cartilaginous intervertebral discs. If osteophytes form, they may press on nerve roots causing neurological symptoms such as numbness and pain into the arm. If the osteophytes are more centrally located, they might lead to spinal stenosis. Although stenosis is less common in the neck than the lumbar spine, the implications are more serious

as long-term neurological complications can arise. These clients must seek medical attention immediately.

Spondylosis, also known as disc degeneration, shows disc changes such as decreased water content, annular tears, collapse, and narrowed disc space. Osteophytes form around the vertebral bodies and there is vertebral body sclerosis (hardening).

Interestingly, many people over the age of thirty show degenerative changes as described making it difficult to differentiate between disease and normal aging. Furthermore, changes seen on an X-ray may not correlate to the symptoms being presented which is why clinicians won't always rush to suggest imaging.

Presentation: The client will complain of stiffness, neck pain that is often a dull ache in the neck radiating to the shoulders and muscle spasm. The pain may refer down into the arm if there are osteophytes pressing on the nerve roots.

Management: Pain relief, warmth, physiotherapy and exercise.

Pilates programme for **degenerative joint disease: osteoarthritis and spondylosis**	Mobilise the neck and thoracic spine gradually with gentle stretches and strengthen the surrounding musculature particularly neck flexors. Work to strengthen the shoulder stabilisers and core muscles to improve overall posture. Support head with cushion when lying supine to achieve correct positioning of head.
Contraindications/ cautions	(Depending on posture) Cervical extension (tipping head back), that is, shortening of neck extensors.

Exercises recommended	Chapter	Exercise no.	Page no.
• Neck exercises on soft ball	9	32, 33	128, 129
• Chin dips seated	9	31	127
• Bug exercise	8	5	93
• Plough	9	17	109
• Cossack seated	13	75	172
• Dart	12	63	160
• Arrow	12	65	161

2. Whiplash

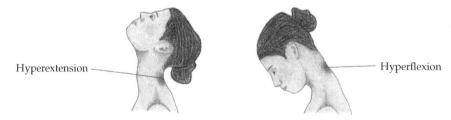

Hyperextension

Hyperflexion

Figure 16. Whiplash.

This term describes bony or soft tissue injuries of the neck that are frequently sustained during car accidents. Classically there is a rear-end collision where the passenger's head jolts backwards but it can also be due to side impact collisions of other activities that mimic this mechanism of injury. There is sudden hyperextension of the lower cervical spine, sometimes with hyperflexion and rotation.

Presentation: Neck pain and stiffness develops usually over the initial 24–48 hours. Other symptoms can include headaches, and radiating neurological signs, jaw pain, tinnitus, and blurred vision. The pattern of recovery is variable with the majority of clients finding that symptoms settle within a few weeks. Factors that might lead to long-term symptoms are increased age, initial severity of symptoms and pre-existing disc degeneration.

Management: Pain relief, warmth, reassurance, encouragement of self-care, to resume normal activities as soon as possible, possible physiotherapy referral for manual techniques and a graded exercise programme. Immobilisation, for example in a soft collar, is not generally recommended. Psychology referral may be appropriate if there are psychological factors to consider such as low expectation of recovery.

Early active exercises are encouraged with work on gentle postural neck exercises and deep neck flexor strengthening. We want to start mobilising the cervical spine within the limits of pain; initially positions that "off-load" the neck such as semi-supine will be most comfortable. In addition, we want to strengthen the muscles around the neck in a way that will not cause further strain and discomfort and start stretching any tight muscles.

Pilates programme for **whiplash**	Mobilise the cervical spine gently in semi-supine and keep the head supported where necessary to achieve the proper alignment of head. Work on strengthening the neck flexors and stretching any surrounding muscles that appear tight. Don't attempt sit-ups or any exercises that will put strain on the neck until strengthened and then support the neck with hands or a folded towel.
Contraindications/ cautions:	Avoid sit-ups until abdominals are strengthened to avoid straining neck. Always use a head cushion to maintain correct alignment of head.

Exercises recommended	Chapter	Exercise no.	Page no.
• Chin dips on soft ball	9	32	128
• Arm circles	9	28	122
• Bug exercise	8	5	93
• Dart	12	63	160
• Arrow	12	65	161
• Abdominal exercise with gym ball/roller	8	8	95
• Leg work on reformer	8	9a, 9b, 9c, 9d	96, 98, 99, 100

(Continued)

Progression	Chapter	Exercise no.	Page no.
• Chin dips seated	9	31	127
• Chest lifts supporting neck	10	39	134
• Oblique lifts supporting neck	10	40	135

3. Acute disc prolapse

Disc prolapse in the cervical spine occurs much less frequently than in the lumbar spine with the most affected levels being C5/6 and C6/7. The prolapse can occur due to local strain or injury, or a sudden unguarded flexion and rotation movement. The disc protrudes and presses on nearby structures including the nerve roots.

Presentation: The client usually complains of neck pain, stiffness, and pain that radiates down into one, or less commonly, both arms. They may also complain of other neurological symptoms in the arms such as numbness, weakness, or pins and needles.

Management: Pain relief, physiotherapy, advice to resume normal activities, and reassurance. If symptoms continue for longer than 4–6 weeks or there are neurological symptoms other than pain, then imaging might be used to assess the nerve root compression in case more invasive interventions are needed such as injections for pain, or surgery.

We want to maintain and gently increase ROM and strengthen surrounding musculature and work in accordance with any instructions provided by the physiotherapist.

Pilates programme for **acute disc prolapse**	Work gently on pelvic stabilisation exercises that don't involve any spinal flexion and strengthen the neck carefully in prone position. Gently increase ROM while strengthening surrounding musculature.
Contraindications/ cautions:	Avoid flexion of the neck. If the person has severe or progressive motor weakness, or severe or progressive sensory loss, seek immediate specialist advice. Use a head cushion to maintain correct alignment whilst in prone position.

Exercises recommended	Chapter	Exercise no.	Page no.
• Dart	12	63	160
• Arrow	12	65	161
• Static abs	8	1	91
• Leg slides	8	4	93
• Abdominal exercise with gym ball/roller	8	8	95
• Arm circles	9	28	122
• Leg work on reformer	8	9a, 9b, 9c, 9d	96, 98, 99, 100

4. Torticollis

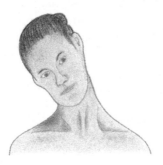

Figure 17. Torticollis.

A torticollis is a painful twisted and tilted neck and is also known as a wry neck. The head is generally tilted to one side and rotated to the other. Onset can be acute, meaning it comes on quickly, for example if the client wakes up with a stiff and painful neck and thinks they might have slept in an awkward position, but often the exact nature of the cause is hard to define. In these situations, symptoms usually ease after 24–48 hours. If the condition doesn't ease the client should see a doctor to try to establish the cause.

Torticollis can sometimes occur after a specific injury, arthritis, or disc prolapse and in such cases the client should be managed by a relevant healthcare professional until an ongoing exercise programme such as Pilates is deemed appropriate.

Presentation: Stiffness, pain, muscle spasm.

Management: Pain relief, warmth, ROM exercises.

Pilates programme for **torticollis**	Gently introduce range of movement exercises for the neck. Strengthen and stabilise the shoulder girdle and stretch any surrounding tight muscles.
Contraindications/ cautions:	Avoid stretching muscles of the neck whilst in spasm, work within pain limits, especially when still very acute.

Exercises recommended	Chapter	Exercise no.	Page no.
• Chin dips on soft ball	9	32	128
• Head rolls on soft ball	9	33	129
• Neck stretch	15	94	195
• Seated plough	9	17	109
• Serratus cushion squeeze	9	21	114
• Dart	12	63	160
• Diamond press	12	64	160
• Arrow	12	65	161

It is useful to be aware that there is another type of torticollis, known as spasmodic torticollis. This type is due to cervical dystonia and is neurological in origin, and presents with uncontrolled movement and muscle spasm. Such cases are managed medically by specialist doctors and physiotherapists, Pilates instructors cannot specifically improve or change this condition. If these clients were to attend for general Pilates it is important that they see a physiotherapist first, preferably one who has Pilates experience, so that they can guide you as to which neck exercises are suitable and those that should be avoided.

5. Cervicogenic headaches

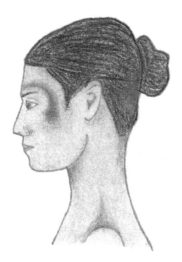

Figure 18. Cervicogenic headaches.

Headaches are classified as primary or secondary. Primary headaches are those that are not a result of another disorder with examples being migraines or tension type headaches. Secondary headaches are as a result of another disorder and cervicogenic headaches (CGH) fall into this category. CGH are headaches that originate from the upper cervical spine due to muscle imbalance that subsequently leads to local joint and soft tissue irritation causing pain to be referred to the head. This muscle imbalance might be as a consequence of injury such as whiplash or, as we commonly see in the Pilates studio, postural issues such as the sustained postures of long hours at a computer or cycling. The important deep postural muscles of the neck become fatigued and overcompensation of the more superficial neck extensors results as they try to hold the head up.

CGH are mostly likely to be seen in people between the ages of thirty and forty-four years with males and females being affected equally. If the headaches are not obviously aggravated by certain neck movements, it is unlikely that their origin is the cervical spine. Primary headaches such as migraines and tension-type headaches (TTH) can also be associated with neck pain and it is important that before starting a Pilates programme, the headache is properly categorised so that it can be managed appropriately.

Presentation: The client usually complains of a unilateral pain of the neck and occiput that can spread to the forehead, jaw line, back of the eyes, and ears. The pain is associated with specific neck movements or sustained postures. There may be reduced cervical spine ROM with increased tightness and overactivity of the anterior and posterior neck muscles.

Management: Physiotherapy that can include techniques such as acupuncture, advice and exercise, balance therapy, and soft tissue massage.

It is important to be aware that patients with migraines and TTH can also complain of neck pain but hopefully by the time they come to Pilates CGH should have been established as the cause. If there are any concerns, then the client should return to their doctor or physiotherapist.

Pilates programme for **cervicogenic headaches**	Retrain the postural muscles of the neck and relax and stretch any muscles that have been overworking and become tight. Work on any postural issues for the whole body particularly scapular positioning and stabilisation.
Contraindications/ cautions	Neck extension initially.

Exercises recommended for cervicogenic headaches	Chapter	Exercise no.	Page no.
• Chin dips on soft ball	9	32	128
• Head rolls on soft ball	9	33	129
• Dart	12	63	160
• Neck stretch	15	94	195
• Seated plough	9	17	109
• Dumb waiter	9	16	107
• Serratus cushion squeeze	9	21	114
• Pectoral stretch	15	90	191
Progression			
• Chin dips seated	9	31	127
• Diamond press	12	64	160
• Serratus exercise on trapeze	9	25	118
• Shoulder mobilisation with TheraBand	9	29	124
• Shoulder mobilisation on trapeze	9	30	126

CHAPTER FOUR

Common conditions of the shoulder

Relevant anatomy and movement
  Common conditions:

1. Rotator cuff disorders
2. Frozen shoulder (adhesive capsulitis)
3. Shoulder dislocation or subluxation (partial dislocation)
4. Winging of the scapula and scapula dyskinesis
5. Osteoarthritis of the glenohumeral joint

Anatomical structure of the shoulder joint

The shoulder or pectoral girdle is made up of a system of bones, joints, and muscles that are designed to support and allow movement of the arm in a free and efficient away in order for us to perform many of the functions of daily life. This is a very mobile joint in comparison to its lower body counterpart, the pelvis and hip where stability is of more importance than mobility.

  The bones that make up the pectoral girdle are the scapula, the humerus, and the clavicle. The joints between these bones are the glenohumeral joint between the glenoid fossa of the scapula, the acromioclavicular joint between the acromion process of the scapula and the clavicle, and the sternoclavicular joint, between the sternum and the clavicle. Sometimes the meeting between the scapular and the thorax is considered as a joint (the scapulothoracic joint) even though two bones do not directly meet. This is because important movement takes place here, which will be discussed later. The anatomy of the shoulder girdle is complex and is only briefly

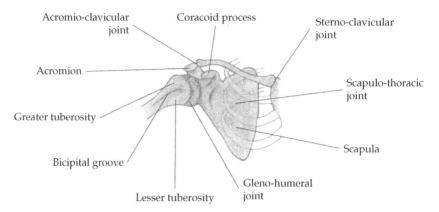

Figure 19. Shoulder joint (anterior view).

visited here so we recommend you visit more in-depth anatomy texts to help with your understanding.

The clavicle can be thought of as a strut that holds the arm away from the body. The small synovial plane acromioclavicular and sternoclavicular joints provide only a little movement and are strengthened by several small ligaments. The glenohumeral joint is a synovial ball and socket joint between the head of the humerus and the glenoid fossa of the scapula. The head of the humerus is much larger in relation to its socket (the glenoid fossa) which allows for a wider range of movement as the head rolls in this socket, which is the opposite to the hip joint where the socket is much larger than the head, making it much more stable for the substantial weight bearing that it has to withstand. Several ligaments provide further stability and so too does the capsule that covers the joint although it should be noted that the capsule is loose inferiorly to allow movement. Several fluid-filled sacs or bursae can be found around the glenohumeral joint that provide cushioning and reduce friction between tendons and bones.

Movements and muscles of the shoulder girdle and shoulder joint

The muscular system of the shoulder girdle is complex, and it is not within the scope of this book to present this in detail, so it is worth referring to further anatomy texts. We will consider the muscles of the shoulder girdle in two groups:

First, the muscles that work to cause movement of the shoulder (glenohumeral) joint. Some of these muscles may only work weakly to move the joint whilst others help by preventing unwanted movement. The four rotator cuff muscles which are named supraspinatous, infraspinatous, teres minor, and subscapularis cause movement of the shoulder but they also stabilise the head of the humerus in the glenoid fossa during movement. Their tendons form a "cuff" around the shoulder joint and in so doing help to reinforce the capsule which assists in preventing dislocation of the joint.

Second, we have muscles that move or stabilise the scapula. These muscles are concerned with stabilising and controlling movement of the scapular which allows efficient glenohumeral movement and subsequently many functional arm activities.

Muscles of the shoulder joint

Approximate full ROM is noted in brackets, as starting from the anatomical position where the person is standing in a neutral position with arms down by their sides, with the palms facing forwards.

Flexion: (180 degrees), deltoid and pectoralis major, biceps, and possibly coracobrachialis.

Extension: (40 degrees), deltoid, teres major, latissimus dorsi, triceps brachii.

Abduction: (160–180 degrees), deltoid, supraspinatus (initiates abduction).

Adduction: (60 degrees), pectoralis major, teres major, latissimus dorsi, teres minor, coracobrachialis, triceps brachii.

Medial rotation: (90 degrees), subscapularis, pectoralis major, latissimus dorsi, teres major, deltoid.

Lateral rotation: (70 degrees), infraspinatus, teres minor, deltoid, pectoralis major.

Muscles that move and stabilise the scapula

Elevation: Upper fibres of trapezius, levator scapulae.
Depression: Lower fibres of trapezius.
Protraction: Serratus anterior
Retraction: Rhomboids, levator scapulae.

Scapulohumeral rhythm

The scapula and the humerus have to move in harmony with one another in order to allow the various movements of the glenohumeral joint with smooth interplay between the many muscles of this area, which then enables efficient upper limb and hand function. Remember also that the design of the joint is such that the glenoid fossa is quite small in relation to the head of the humerus; the head of the humerus can move and roll around the glenoid fossa in many different ways. Correct position of the scapula provides suitable alignment of the glenoid fossa which should be directed superior-medially so that it can join with the head of the humerus without impingement of nearby soft tissue structures. To enable this alignment, the ideal position for the scapula on the posterior thorax should be over the second to seventh ribs with a rotation of approximately thirty degrees anteriorly from the frontal plane. As we move the humerus for various arm functions, the scapula must glide smoothly over the muscles and ribs so that the glenoid fossa orientation can change to match the position of the humerus. If everything is working in harmony risk of common injuries, for example, impingement (or pinching) to the shoulder joint structures such as the rotator cuff tendons or bursae, are minimised. This is often referred to as a good scapula-humeral rhythm, that is, the two bones are moving well in relation to each other so as to achieve a good range of movement and function that is pain-free. A good scapula-humeral rhythm is particularly pertinent when considering large movements of the shoulder such as abduction and flexion. In the first sixty degrees of shoulder flexion and thirty degrees of shoulder abduction the movement of the scapula is variable, and this is known as the setting phase. After this initial phase, for every two degrees of glenohumeral movement there is one degree of scapula movement although exact measures are likely to vary.

If we think about shoulder abduction, to begin with most movement occurs only at the glenohumeral joint with supraspinatus initiating the first twenty degrees of movement to achieve correct position of the humerus in order for deltoid to take over. As we said before the other rotator cuff muscles are also activated in order to stabilise the head of the humerus in the glenoid fossa. For full abduction the shoulder should be gently rotated laterally to start with, which clears the head of the humerus from the acromion process of the scapula and will prevent impingement. The stabilising muscles of the scapula allow for it to move smoothly without "hitching up" which also helps reduce the chance of impingement. In the Pilates studio we often ask our clients to "draw the shoulder blades down the back" or to "not let the shoulders shrug up" as they perform exercises such as arm circles.

Let us imagine that the scapula wasn't able to move during arm movement so that the glenoid fossa position couldn't change according to the needs of the task: functional activities would be so much more difficult. For example, brushing your hair, doing up your bra strap, reaching forwards, pushing a heavy object forward, swimming, or pushing on the arms of a chair as you stand up. Imagine these activities without the smooth interplay between the scapulothoracic and glenohumeral joints, or if the scapula was not designed to move.

It is also important to remember how posture affects the position of the shoulder girdle and arm movement. You can feel this by sitting in a chair and slumping down into trunk flexion; from there try to fully elevate your arm through flexion or abduction. The ROM is considerably less than if you do this while sitting up nice and straight. This gentle extension needs to be of the thoracic spine and not just an overarching of the lumbar spine.

Common conditions

Be aware that pain in the shoulder or arm can sometimes be referred from the neck but hopefully this will have been established by a medical or healthcare professional. As we have discussed, good posture is so important for correct shoulder girdle alignment and it always needs to be considered when working with clients with shoulder issues. In turn, good shoulder stability is required in order to achieve good arm ROM and effective, pain-free function.

1. Rotator cuff disorders
Rotator cuff disorders refer to rotator cuff tendinopathy or any pain or pathology associated with the rotator cuff tendons and include partial or full tears. Rotator cuff pathology leads to subacromial shoulder pain which is felt on top of the shoulder

and laterally and is the commonest cause of shoulder pain seen in people between the ages of thirty-five and seventy-five. The rotator cuff tendons can be injured by a traumatic incident (usually in young to middle age), such as a fall or accident, or more commonly by wear and tear and inflammation over a long time. If the cause isn't addressed, then eventually there may be a partial or complete tear of one of more of the rotator cuff tendons. Rotator cuff tendinopathy is also known as impingement because there is usually impingement or "pinching" of the tendons between bony structures. If we refer to Figure 19 we will see that the rotator cuff tendons sit under the coracoacromial arch and insert into the greater tubercle of the humerus. The arch is made up of bone and ligaments and there is also a subacromial bursa here to aid friction-free movement. Because this bursa can also get inflamed leading to subacromial bursitis it is also included under the umbrella of impingement or rotator cuff tendinopathy.

Impingement can occur for several reasons: some people may have a naturally small subacromial space or osteoarthritis with osteophyte formation may add to this space being smaller. Sometimes impingement can occur due to overuse if a person's occupation or sport is one that involves repetitive overhead action, for example, painter/decorator or javelin thrower. In these circumstances we refer to primary impingement.

Shoulder instability, inactivity, and poor posture can all lead to imbalance of the muscles that move and stabilise the shoulder girdle, which will alter the position of the scapula and result in narrowing of the subacromial space. As a result, the shoulder girdle is not positioned in the right place leaving the rotator cuff muscles having to work extra hard to stabilise the head of the humerus in the shoulder joint. Eventually the muscles fatigue and can no longer hold the head of the humerus down, resulting in secondary impingement and inflammation of the tendons.

Presentation: Pain is felt on the top of the shoulder and laterally and increases with lifting, for example a heavy kettle, or overhead activities, such as painting a high wall or overarm throwing during sporting activities. The client may report pain at night. Clinicians sometimes check for a painful arc which refers to pain between

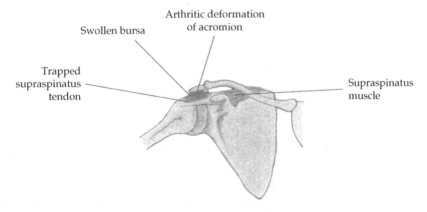

Figure 20. Shoulder impingement (anterior view).

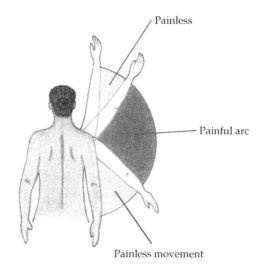

Painless

Painful arc

Painless movement

**Shoulder impingement
(painful arc) syndrome**

Figure 21. Shoulder impingement and painful arc.

70–120 degrees of abduction; in this range the subacromial structures are in closer contact with the surrounding bony structures than they are at the start and end of abduction. Pain on abduction may be worse with the thumb down as this places the shoulder in medial rotation. If we abduct with the thumb facing up (where shoulder is now in lateral rotation) the greater tubercle is cleared from the subacromial arch, decreasing the risk of impingement.

Traumatic tears usually present with extreme pain and weakness and it is important that these are diagnosed as soon as possible as delay in diagnosis can adversely affect the success of surgical repair.

Management: Initially the client will be advised to rest but they should not stop moving their arm for a prolonged period and immobilisation in a sling is not recommended. Simple pain relief and ice can help to alleviate pain and they may be referred to physiotherapy. Sometimes the doctor will recommend a steroid injection to help with pain. If the situation does not improve surgery can be considered to widen the subacromial space and if the client comes to Pilates after surgery it is important to follow the post-operative guidelines and advice from the hospital and physiotherapist.

If the client has seen a physiotherapist be guided by any advice that they have been given. Generally, you will want to have a look at the posture and think about how it might be affecting the alignment of the shoulder girdle. If there is evidence of an upper crossed syndrome (see Chapter Seven) this should be addressed. Concentrate on improving stability and motor control around the whole shoulder girdle, particularly the lower trapezius, latissimus dorsi, and serratus anterior, with the aim to correctly align the glenoid fossa. This will hopefully reduce the amount of impinge-ment of the tendons within the subacromial space. Regarding shoulder ROM, ini-tially work within a pain-free range, perhaps starting with static exercises. We want to strengthen the rotator cuff muscles in a graded way, in other words, gradually increas-ing the resistance as pain diminishes.

Pilates programme for **rotator cuff injuries**	Work to stabilise the shoulder girdle and address any postural issues such as upper crossed syndrome. Strengthen the main shoulder stabilisers (lower trapezius, serratus anterior, and latissimus dorsi) initially with closed chain exercises. Start to increase ROM when pain-free and strengthen rotator cuff muscles gradually, only adding resistance when able to hold form.
Contraindications/ cautions:	Overhead arm movements until they have great motor control and stability around the shoulder girdle and less pain.

Exercises recommended	Chapter	Exercise no.	Page no.
• Seated plough	9	17	109
• Serratus cushion squeeze	9	21	114
• Arm lifts	9	19	112
• Standing arm lift against wall	9	20	113
• Dumb waiter	9	16	107
Progression			
• Dumb waiter with TheraBand	9	16a	108
• Serratus exercise on trapeze	9	25	118
• Dumb waiter on reformer	9	16b	108
• Seated plough on reformer	9	18	111
• Shoulder mobilisation with push through bar on trapeze	9	30	126

2. Frozen shoulder (adhesive capsulitis)

The pathology of a frozen shoulder is poorly understood but is generally defined by adhesions and contractures of the fibrous capsule of the glenohumeral joint. It is a common condition that causes pain and stiffness with a progressive loss of active and passive shoulder movement. It is most frequently seen in people aged forty to sixty and is more common in women than men and those that have previously had a frozen shoulder of the opposite arm. This condition can be primary, occurring spontaneously, or it can be secondary and associated with trauma, diabetes, thyroid conditions, hemi-plegia (weakness of the arm after a stroke) and cardiovascular disease. Symptoms usually settle within eighteen to twenty-four months although some people report ongoing pain and stiffness for several years.

Presentation: There tends to be three overlapping phases:

1) The painful phase whereby the shoulder gradually becomes stiff and painful, in the deltoid area causing discomfort day and night, especially if lying on that side. All movements are restricted but particularly external rotation. Activities such as brushing hair, putting on a jacket or fastening a bra strap become difficult. This phase tends to last several months.
2) The stiffness phase which can last up to a year with sustained stiffness and little range of movement, but pain will subside. Function continues to be significantly impaired.
3) The resolution phase shows gradual improvement as the shoulder starts to regain movement and this phase may last from one to three years.

Management: The client will be offered reassurance that despite stiffness worsening in the first stages this will gradually resolve. Pain relief can be taken as necessary; use of heat packs, supporting the arm in bed with pillows, and avoiding rolling onto this side at night can be advised. They should also be encouraged to use and move the arm as much as possible within the limits of pain. They may be offered physiotherapy for exercise programmes and pain relief modalities. If symptoms don't improve steroid injections can be considered and referral to orthopaedics if they have had substantial pain and stiffness for up to three months and no improvement with conservative measures.

Pilates can be offered at any stage of having a frozen shoulder, but we want to work within the limits of pain, especially during the early stages, aiming to maintain and improve ROM of the glenohumeral joint as much as is possible. In addition to this it is important to work on scapula stability and motor control and to also consider posture (particularly in the thoracic area) and the effect that any postural dysfunction might have on scapula and shoulder joint alignment.

Pilates programme for frozen shoulder **(adhesive capsulitis)**	Work to improve posture particularly around the thoracic area whilst improving ROM and stability of the shoulder girdle.
Contraindications/ cautions:	Do not stop moving the shoulder but keep within range of comfort.

Exercises recommended	*Chapter*	*Exercise no.*	*Page no.*
• Cossack arms (semi supine)	9	27	121
• Lift and lower with stick	9	19	112
• Serratus cushion squeeze	9	21	114
• Seated plough	9	17	109
• Dumb waiter	9	16	107
• Shoulder rehab; arm slide and lift on bench	9	26	120
• Shoulder joint release Prone on bed " (or forward leaning) single arm circles	9	34	130

3. Shoulder instability

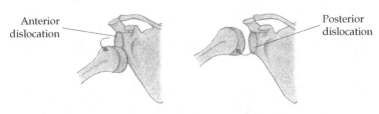

Figure 22. Shoulder dislocation.

As we said earlier, the shoulder joint has sacrificed stability for mobility where the head of the humerus is large in relation to the glenoid fossa in which it sits. Through this design the head of the humerus can move or roll around the glenoid fossa resulting in a large ROM that affords us many different functional activities. The downside is that the shoulder is more at risk of instability or dislocation (usually anteriorly). When shoulder instability occurs the movement between the joint surfaces, that is, the head of the humerus and glenoid fossa, is dysfunctional causing pain, subluxation (partial loss of contact between the joint surfaces), or dislocation (complete loss of contact between the surfaces). Dislocation can be acute, happening as one-off, recurrent, or locked. Sometimes clients may have joint laxity without symptoms. This is when there is increased movement of the head of the humerus within the glenoid fossa at the upper end of the normal shoulder ROM. Joint laxity and instability can occur together, or they can exist as separate entities.

Shoulder instability is classified as the following:

- Traumatic, whereby the shoulder is dislocated by an external force, for example during contact sports, and if shoulder structures do not heal with the shoulder in the correct alignment, recurrent dislocation is likely.
- Atraumatic instability is most common in teenage girls who have hypermobility (increased joint mobility and laxity). This makes the shoulder joint more prone to instability following a minor injury or sometimes with no preceding event.
- Instability due to poor muscle patterning. This is where there is no abnormality of shoulder joint structures and the cause is actually muscle imbalance often due to postural dysfunction, for example, with the upper crossed syndrome.

Prolonged instability can be associated with osteoarthritis due to long-term malalignment of the joint surfaces.

Presentation: Shoulder instability usually occurs in people who are aged thirty-five years or under. It may be that they have a few non-specific symptoms such as clicking, pain. or an ache, or they report a feeling of the shoulder partially or completely coming out of place. They may feel apprehensive that it will occur during certain activities or sports. Sometimes, if the instability has been present for a prolonged length of time, nerves can be affected leading to symptoms in the arm and hand such as tingling and numbness. Beware the client who describes "popping" their shoulder out of joint and putting it back in as a party trick!

Traumatic dislocation, which is usually in an anterior direction due to the anatomical design of the glenohumeral joint, is most common in younger people, frequently during contact sports, or women over the age of eighty who fall on an outstretched arm. During the traumatic incident other damage may occur such as nerve damage, humeral fracture, or a rotator cuff tear. A posterior shoulder dislocation is less common than an anterior one but can be sustained during a seizure so must be considered if there is shoulder pain after such an event.

Management: For traumatic, acute dislocations and associated fractures medical management is essential, initially in Accident & Emergency, as the joint (and bone if there is a fracture) needs to be repositioned through manipulation or sometimes surgery. After this, substantial physiotherapy will be required for careful mobilisation and strengthening. The healthcare professionals will also be mindful of the possibility of shoulder instability and rotator cuff damage. Recurrent dislocations, associated fractures, posterior dislocations after seizures, or those who have had a one-off dislocation but are negatively impacted by ongoing symptoms should all be seen by a shoulder surgeon.

Atraumatic instability due to poor muscle patterning requires a referral to physiotherapy, or if that is of no benefit then referral to orthopaedics is indicated.

For all joint instability early mobilisation after initial medical management is encouraged and should be within the limits of pain. Physiotherapy works on maintaining the position of the relocation allowing the surrounding structures to heal. Therapists will address any postural issues or muscle imbalance and work on muscle activation that promotes stability.

It is really important to work in line with advice as set out by the doctors and physiotherapists in order to avoid further instability or dislocation. It might be that some movements are to be avoided in the first few days and weeks and it is vital that this information is gathered before Pilates instructors start working with the client. Once the relevant information and advice from the healthcare professionals is acquired, work on improving stability and motor control of the muscles that work around the scapula, and improve posture and alignment which will allow more efficient muscle activation through achieving optimum muscle length. Hopefully, this will help to attain a more stable base from which the glenohumeral joint can work effectively. Only then start to gently increase ROM of the glenohumeral joint and increase the strength of the rotator cuff muscles and other muscles that act to move the shoulder.

Pilates programme for **shoulder dislocation or subluxation** (partial dislocation) and general shoulder instability (hypermobility)	Work to stabilise the shoulder girdle and strengthen the surrounding musculature such as rotator cuff muscles. In order to do this, make sure there is good core strength already in place. Keep to closed chain exercises if hypermobility is present in the shoulder joint.
Contraindications/cautions:	Exercise only when instructed by physiotherapist.

Recommended exercises	Chapter	Exercise no.	Page no.
• Arm lifts	9	19	112
• Serratus cushion squeeze	9	21	114
• Seated plough	9	17	109
• Dumb waiter	9	16	107
• Standing arm lift against wall	9	20	113
• Supine serratus exercise with springs on trapeze	9	25	118
• Shoulder rehab exercise (slide and lift on bench)	9	26	120
• Deltoid arm lifts	9	23	116
• Superman (arm lifts only)	12	69	166

Progression			
• Dumb waiter with TheraBand	9	16a	108
• Serratus exercise with TheraBand kneeling	9	22	114
• Serratus exercise with TheraBand supine	9	24	117
• Supine shoulder mobilisation with TheraBand	9	29	124
• Supine shoulder mobilisation with push through bar on trapeze	9	30	126
• Plough on reformer	9	18	111
• Dumb waiter on reformer	9	16b	108
• Serratus exercise on reformer	9	22a	114
• Kneeling plank on reformer	8	13	104

4. Winging of the scapula and scapula dyskinesis

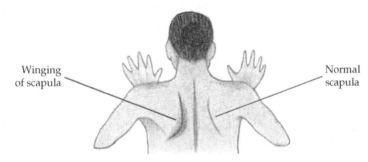

Figure 23. Winging scapula.

Winging of the scapula is, in simple terms, where we see part of the scapula protruding posteriorly, and scapula dyskinesis refers to the abnormal movement patterns of the scapula that can result in this winging. The incorrect position of the scapula can result in pain, decreased ROM, and further disruption in harmonious scapulo-humeral rhythm, all of which will have a knock-on effect on arm function. Although a winging scapula is a common term that is used frequently in Pilates practice, it is in fact a quite complex phenomenon with several causes beyond simple muscle imbalance.

To very briefly recap: the scapula is a flat bone with many different stability and mobility muscles attached to it and it is really important that all these muscles work together in harmony to allow smooth shoulder girdle movement and good function of the arm. If, for whatever reason these muscles are not working as a team we may see poor scapulohumeral rhythm, or scapula dyskinesis, and winging of the scapula can be just one manifestation of this problem. Scapula dyskinesis can *cause* further shoulder pathologies or it can *be caused* by shoulder pathologies. If it is concluded that factors within and around the shoulder joint are the cause of the winging, such as glenohumeral instability, damage within the joint or perhaps pathology of the acromioclavicular joint, it is imperative that this is addressed by a doctor or healthcare professional such as a physiotherapist in case expert management is required.

Winging can also be caused by damage to the nerve that supplies serratus anterior, damage to the trapezius and rhomboid muscles, or might be associated with certain muscular dystrophies. In these situations, we strongly advise that you work with these clients as guided by the medics and physiotherapists. Generally, these circumstances will be uncommon in daily practice and the winging that you are likely to come across will be due to muscle imbalance as a result of postural dysfunction or shoulder pathologies.

When working with a winging scapular or scapular dyskinesis it is worth revisiting the anatomy of the shoulder musculature and to particularly remember that the job of serratus anterior is to keep the scapula close to the thorax. Another thing to look out for is when only the inferior angle of the scapula protrudes which is usually due to tightness of the pectoralis minor muscle. Pectoralis minor attaches to the coracoid process at the front of the scapula and if it is tight it can pull and rotate the top of the scapula anteriorly resulting in protrusion of the inferior angle.

Presentation: There will be a winged scapula and/or a dysfunctional movement pattern as we have described above, possibly associated with other factors such as a shoulder pathology or muscular dystrophy or more simply with a postural dysfunction.

Management: This will depend on the cause and whether the client is involved with specialist doctors or physiotherapists. Once the cause is established management can vary from exercise and movement rehabilitation with the physiotherapists, to surgery.

Our general aims are to improve any faulty scapulohumeral rhythm and address any muscle imbalance issues that we find. We do this through scapula setting exercises, specific Pilates scapula mobility and strengthening exercises, and then combining scapula stability with shoulder ROM exercises. If there is associated shoulder pathology that might be contributing to the winging or dyskinesis such as a rotator cuff disorder or frozen shoulder, then remember to individualise your programme accordingly.

Pilates programme for **winging of the scapula and scapula dyskinesis**	Address any postural muscle imbalances particularly around the shoulder girdle. Work to stabilise and strengthen the serratus anterior and stretch the pectoral muscles particularly pec minor.
Contraindications/ cautions:	Avoid weight loading exercises (planks etc.) until serratus is strengthened.

Exercises recommended	Chapter	Exercise no.	Page no.
• Serratus cushion squeeze	9	21	114
• Standing arm lift against wall	9	20	113
• Serratus exercise with TheraBand kneeling	9	22	114
• Serratus exercise with TheraBand supine	9	24	117
• Shoulder mobilisation with push through bar on trapeze	9	30	126
• Serratus exercise on reformer	9	22a	114
• Dumb waiter on reformer	9	16b	108
• Supine serratus exercise on trapeze	9	25	118
• Pectoral stretch on roller	15	92	192
• Around the world stretch	15	93	193
• Arm circles	9	28	122

5. Arthritis of the glenohumeral joint

We have briefly mentioned osteoarthritis in relation to the cervical and lumbar spine areas, and later on when we cover the hip and knee, we go into more detail of the degenerative changes that occur with this condition. Although osteoarthritis occurs more frequently in the increased weight-bearing joints (hence why we go into more detail in the relevant chapters) any synovial joint is susceptible, and we see a number of clients with shoulder joint arthritis at our studios.

Presentation: The client may complain of joint stiffness with decreased ROM, pain, and difficulty with everyday functions such as getting their arm in and out of clothes and doing their hair.

Management: The clinicians will consider the severity of symptoms and how the person is affected in regard to function and quality of life. Management options include education and advice; exercise and physiotherapy referral; occupational therapy for assistive devices; pain relief; steroid injection. Surgery might be considered if symptoms don't improve with conservative management.

Pilates programme for **arthritis of the glenohumeral joint**	Address any muscle imbalances around the shoulder girdle. Work to strengthen the musculature around the joint and improve range of movement.
Contraindications/cautions:	Do not exercise when the joint is inflamed.

Exercises recommended	Chapter	Exercise no.	Page no.
• Cossack arms supine	9	27	121
• Shoulder rehab exercise; arm slide and lift on bench	9	26	120
• Serratus cushion squeeze	9	21	114
• Arm lifts	9	19	112

(Continued)

Exercises recommended	Chapter	Exercise no.	Page no.
• Dumb waiter	9	16	107
• Seated plough	9	17	109
• Serratus exercise on trapeze	9	25	118
• Shoulder joint release	9	34	130

Progression			
• Standing arm lift	9	20	113
• Arm circles	9	28	122
• Shoulder mobilisation with TheraBand	9	29	124
• Shoulder mobilisation with push through bar on trapeze	9	30	126

CHAPTER FIVE

Common conditions of the pelvis and hip

Relevant anatomy and movement
   Conditions:

1. Greater trochanteric pain syndrome (GTPS), previously trochanteric bursitis
2. Sacroiliac dysfunction
3. Piriformis syndrome
4. Iliopsoas syndrome
5. Groin (adductor) strain
6. Osteitis pubis
7. Osteoarthritis of the hip and hip replacements

Anatomy of the pelvis and hip

The pelvic girdle

The pelvic girdle or pelvis is a basin-shaped ring of bone consisting of the right and left hip bones that meet at the front via the pubic symphysis joint and at the back via the sacrum and two joints. Each hip bone is made up of three bones: the ilium, ischium, and pubic bone which fuse together after puberty. The pelvic girdle is strong and rigid compared to the mobile shoulder girdle, this being achieved through its anatomical design and complex of strong muscles and ligaments. Without this stability there would be a detrimental increased load through the hips, knees, and feet leading to pain and dysfunction.

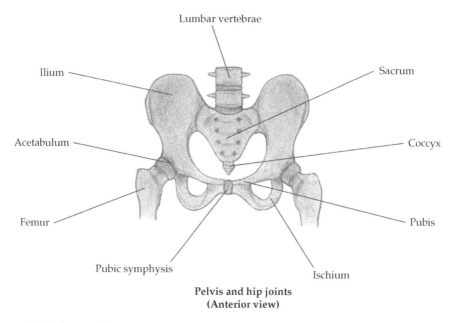

Pelvis and hip joints
(Anterior view)

Figure 24. Pelvis and hip joints.

The male and female pelvis differ, the most significant difference being in shape where the male pelvis is more heart-shaped and deep compared to the rounder, shallower female pelvis which aids childbirth. Further functions of the pelvis are:

- To provide connection between the vertebral column and the femurs
- To provides subtle joint movement that assists correct lower limb movement
- Transfer of the weight of the axial skeleton to the lower limbs when sitting, standing, and walking
- To support and protect the pelvic organs
- To provide attachment for powerful muscles.

The hip

The hip is a synovial ball and socket joint made up of the acetabulum of the hip bone (the socket) and the head of the femur (the ball). The hip joint has a good ROM while being exceptionally stable, the head of the femur fitting snugly in the relatively deep acetabulum, with further stability provided by strong ligaments and muscles. Both hip joints together, and in conjunction with the pelvic girdle, connect the mass of the trunk to the legs enduring great amounts of weight-bearing so a design that allows for increased stability is very important. Unlike with the shoulder, dislocation is rare except with extreme forces such as during a car crash.

Because of its function, the hip joint is subject to inflammation and degenerative disease, and hence is one of the most common joints to be replaced. The articular surfaces of the joint are the acetabulum of the hip bone and the head of the femur, both of which are covered in smooth hyaline cartilage which aids friction-free movement. The synovial fluid within the joint provides nutrition for this cartilage and cyclical compression triggers increased fluid production. This in turn aids absorption of wear particles and lubricates the joint making weight-bearing through the joint very important.

Like the shoulder joint several bursae can be found around the hip joint which protect other soft tissues from friction forces; for example, the superficial trochanteric bursa which is found on the outside of the hip between the greater trochanter and the ilio-tibial band (ITB).

Movement and muscles of the pelvis and hip joints

Little movement occurs at joints of the pelvis because as previously explained it is designed for stability. This isn't to say that there is no movement at all at these joints: a very small amount of mobility is required at the sacroiliac (SI) joints during everyday function where the pelvis tilts anteriorly, posteriorly, and laterally during movements such as going from sitting to lying, or during walking. The pubic symphysis is mostly immoveable but this changes during pregnancy: hormones act on the ligaments to cause softening which allows more movement thus aiding the birthing process.

With regards to the hip, movement described is actually movement of the thigh on the trunk, not actually movement between the head of the femur and the acetabulum. This is because the shaft of the femur is held away from the head by the neck of the femur. The angle between neck and shaft is approximately 125 degrees. Rotation around the long axis of the neck translates as flexion and extension of the hip.

The movements and muscles of the hip are summarised below, but it is also important that as Pilates instructors we are familiar with all the muscles that attach to pelvis. Some connect to the hip and others connect to the trunk so many of them not only produce movement but also serve to stabilise the pelvis during functions such as walking. It is a good idea to refer to more in-depth anatomy texts to gain a deeper understanding of these muscles.

Flexion: (120 degrees), psoas major, tensor facia lata (TFL), rectus femoris, sartorius, some adductors.

Extension: (15 degrees), gluteus maximus, hamstrings, some adductors.

Abduction: (40 degrees), gluteus medius, gluteus minimus, TFL.

Adduction: Adductors (longus, brevis, and magnus), pectineus, and gracilis.

Medial rotation: TFL, anterior fibres of gluteus medius, gluteus minimus.

Lateral rotation: obturator muscles, gemelli muscles, piriformis, quadratus femoris.

After the specific joint movement occurs, the pelvis and spine then come in to play.

Conditions

1. Greater trochanteric pain syndrome (GTPS)

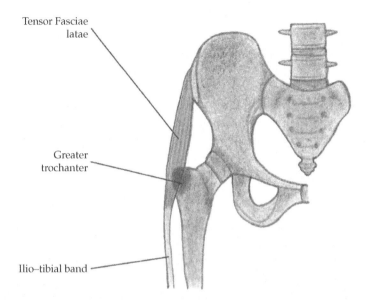

Tensor Fasciae
latae

Greater
trochanter

Ilio–tibial band

Figure 25. Greater trochanteric pain syndrome.

GTPS used to be known as trochanteric bursitis as it was thought that discomfort on the outside of the hip, over the surface of the greater trochanter was caused by inflammation of the trochanteric bursae. However, more recent research has shown that pain in this region might also be due to injury or inflammation of other soft tissue structures such as muscles and tendons (primarily the gluteal tendons), so the broader term, GTPS is used. This syndrome is more common in women than men, particularly those that are obese, and can occur in conjunction with low back pain. Inflammation of the soft tissue structures can be as a result of overuse injuries which can alter biomechanics and muscle balance; for example, in issues with the iliotibial band (ITB); infection; direct injury; tendon damage; leg length discrepancy, or hip surgery such as a total hip replacement.

Presentation: The client will complain of pain on the lateral aspect of the hip in the area of the greater trochanter and this area may be tender to touch. Pain, often described as a deep ache or burning, will be gradual at onset or can start after a specific event. The pain is often aggravated by resisted hip abduction and/or rotation and activities such as climbing stairs, running, walking, or sitting with crossed legs. Lying on the affected side can be uncomfortable, gait pattern can be altered, and hip range of movement may be decreased.

Management: Most people with GTPS will find that their symptoms resolve with time. The doctor will usually advise pain relief and anti-inflammatories as necessary, applying ice and resting from the aggravating activities. Increased body weight should be addressed appropriately. If symptoms are ongoing steroid injections can be offered, or the client can be referred for physiotherapy where assessment and treatment aim to improve the health of the lateral hip soft tissue structures through an exercise and stretching programme and by addressing any postural or biomechanical issues.

Pilates programme for **greater trochanteric pain syndrome (GTPS)**	Stretch the surrounding structures including those of the hip region and lumbar spine. Work out which muscles are tight and which are weak. Usually the hip flexors and deep external rotators tend to be tight and the hip extensors and hip abductors tend to be weak. Address any postural issues and improve standing balance.
Contraindications/cautions	Lying on the affected side can be aggravating so you need to adapt the programme accordingly.

Exercises recommended	Chapter	Exercise no.	Page no.
• Prone gluteal squeeze	11	55	152
• Prone hamstring curls	11	56	152
• Knee lifts	8	7	94
• Leg slides	8	4	93
• Reformer leg work	8	9a, 9b	96, 98
• Prancers	8	10	102
• Hip abduction supine on trapeze	11	51	148
• Small hip rolls	13	73	170
• Piriformis stretch	15	95	195
• Iliopsoas stretch	15	86, 87	188, 189
• Quadriceps stretch	15	85	187
• Buttock stretch	15	90	191
Progression			
• Bug	8	5	93
• Large hip rolls	13	74	171
• Clam*	11	48	145
• Side lying hip exercise*	11	49	146
• Hip abduction exercise*	11	50	147
• Prone hamstring curls with hip extension	11	57	153
• Superman hip extension	12	69	166
• Glute med standing (combo chair)	11	61	157
• Iliopsoas stretch	15	86, 88, 89	188, 190

* If able to lie on side

2. Sacroiliac dysfunction

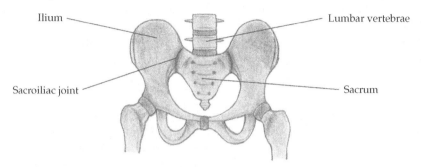

Figure 26. Sacroiliac joint pain.

The SI joint is a common source of low back pain and several processes can lead to its dysfunction, such as degenerative joint disease, trauma, ligament laxity during pregnancy, or malalignment due to muscle imbalance or altered posture, such as scoliosis. The SI joint is formed between the sacrum and the ilium and the joint surface is covered in articular cartilage and bound by strong ligaments. There is only very slight movement forwards and backwards and minimal rotation.

The design of the joint surfaces along with the strong ligaments and surrounding muscles provide the SI joint with great stability but if subjected to any conditions discussed above, this can be reduced, changing biomechanics and joint alignment putting strain on all structures involved which can subsequently lead to pain.

Presentation: A dull ache is felt at the base of the spine usually on the affected side. The pain may become sharp with activities such as sitting, bending, sit to stand, lifting the knee up, as in climbing stairs. Pain can refer to the back, groin, buttock, and the back of the thigh but does not usually radiate below the knee. The referred pain may feel sciatic in nature with the client describing a burning or stabbing pain. If there is any instability of the pelvis there may be a feeling of buckling or giving way. Sometimes there can be inflammation of the joint, also known as sacroiliitis, that can lead to pain and stiffness.

Management: Pain relief and physiotherapy are recommended but if there is little positive effect with these interventions then steroid injections can be considered. If, however, chronic pain continues referral to spinal or orthopaedic surgeons is an option and they will explore with the client various surgical interventions.

Pilates programme for **sacroiliac dysfunction**	Try to strengthen the core (pelvic floor, transversus, multifidus) and stretch surrounding muscles. Gently mobilise the joint if there is any stiffness, as well as addressing any postural issues that may be contributing to poor joint alignment.
Contraindications/cautions:	Avoid spinal extension and hip external rotation initially.

Exercises recommended	Chapter	Exercise no.	Page no.
• Small tilts	10	35	131
• Small tilts on soft ball	10	36	132
• Abdominal exercise with gym ball/roller	8	8	95
• Small hip rolls	13	73	170
• Prone gluteal squeeze	11	55	152
• Curl down (half) with TheraBand	10	41	136
• Chest lifts	10	39	134
• Cat (no extension)	10	43	138
• Lumbar circles	13	72	170
• Lumbar stretch	15	96	196
Progression			
• Prone hamstring curls	11	56	152
• Swimming prep	12	62	159
• Clam	11	48	145
• Tippy toes on soft ball	8	14	105
• Butterfly on soft ball	8	15	106
• Iliopsoas and lumbar stretch on soft ball	15	88	190
• Large hip rolls	13	74	171
• Hip circles with TheraBand	11	53	150
• Hip circles on reformer	11	54	150

3. Piriformis syndrome

Sometimes pain radiating down the leg or "sciatica" is not because of nerve root compression in the lower back as you might think. It might actually be due to the piriformis muscle compressing on and irritating the sciatic nerve as it emerges from the sciatic notch. Why this happens is not clear: it might be as a result of trauma with resulting inflammation and muscle spasm, or it might be due to muscle shortening because of altered biomechanics in the back, pelvis, and hip regions. Overuse may also be a contender, perhaps in long distance walking or running, where repeated microtrauma leads to inflammation and tightness. Piriformis syndrome is more commonly seen in women, perhaps due to the wider pelvis.

Presentation: The client complains of pain in the buttock that can radiate to the hip and down the leg to the foot. There may also be other neurological signs such as pins and needles and numbness. Pain will often be aggravated by activities such as running and walking, prolonged sitting, squatting, hip adduction, and internal rotation. Movements that stretch the piriformis are also likely to be aggravating.

Management: The doctor may suggest that the client takes non-steroidal anti-inflammatories; physiotherapy is recommended to advise on correct stretches, to address biomechanical issues, and possible soft tissue treatment techniques. Steroid injections may be considered.

Pilates programme for	Check posture and alignment and work to gently stretch
Piriformis syndrome	the piriformis but at the same time strengthen the medial hip rotators and hip abductors.
Contraindications/cautions	Excessive use of deep external hip rotators.

Exercises recommended	Chapter	Exercise no.	Page no.
• Parallel leg work on reformer	8	9a, 9b	96, 98
• Side lying hip exercise	11	49	146
• Hip abductor exercise	11	50	147
• Glute med standing (combo chair)	11	61	157
• Piriformis stretch	15	95	195
• Buttock stretch	15	90	191

4. Iliopsoas syndrome

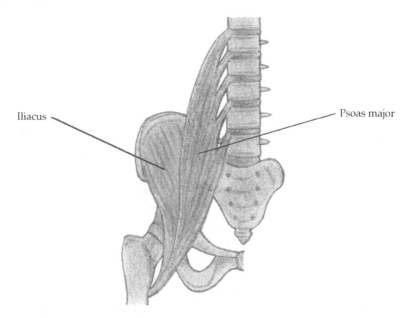

Figure 27. Iliopsoas.

Iliopsoas syndrome refers to inflammation of the hip flexor tendon with or without a bursitis of the iliopsoas bursa. It is commonly caused by overuse or trauma, mostly seen in athletes such as runners, gymnasts, dancers, or footballers. This syndrome can be associated with other musculoskeletal conditions such as arthritis, trauma, and hip replacements. It can also be as a result of repetitive hip flexion activities.

Presentation: Pain is located on the anteromedial aspect of the thigh and can radiate into the leg but not usually below the knee. It will appear during walking or movement such as crossing the legs. Hip flexion, internal rotation, and passive hip extension may elicit pain. Pain increases with the activity and is relieved with rest. The client may complain of stiffness and pain in the morning and sometimes describes a snapping sensation at the front of the hip. There may also be low back pain.

Management: Physiotherapy is recommended to address any muscle imbalance. The doctor may suggest over-the-counter pain relief; sometimes a steroid injection will be considered.

Pilates programme for **Iliopsoas syndrome**	Work to gently balance the strength and tightness of the surrounding muscles. Strengthen the hip extensors to stop the hip flexors overworking and the deep core muscles to ensure neutral spine can be held when necessary and posture improved when standing.
Contraindications/cautions	Wait for pain and inflammation to subside before exercising.

Exercises recommended	Chapter	Exercise no.	Page no.
• Prone gluteal squeeze	11	55	152
• Prone hamstring curls	11	56	152
• Leg slides	8	4	93
• Knee lifts	8	7	94
• Assisted bridge on trapeze	8	12	103
• Chest lifts	10	39	134
• Mini curl up on trapeze	10	45	140
• Oblique chest lifts	10	40	135
• Abdominal exercise with gym ball/roller	8	8	95
• Iliopsoas stretch standing	15	86	188
• Iliopsoas and lumbar stretch on soft ball	15	88	190
Progression			
• Hamstring exercise on trapeze	11	59	156
• Bridge	8	11	102
• Leg work on reformer	8	9a, 9b, 9c	96, 98, 99
• Superman	12	69	166
• Superman on reformer	12	70	167
• Tippy toes on soft ball	8	14	105
• Iliopsoas stretch on table (Thomas test)	15	87	189
• Psoas stretch on reformer	15	89	190
• Quadriceps stretch	15	85	187

5. Groin (adductor) strain

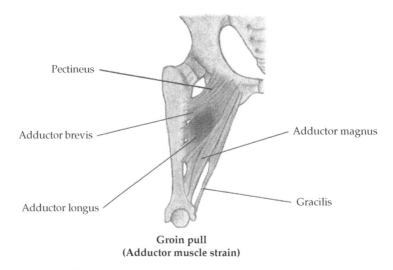

Pectineus

Adductor brevis

Adductor magnus

Adductor longus

Gracilis

Groin pull
(Adductor muscle strain)

Figure 28. Groin (adductor) strain.

This is one of the most common injuries in sports especially those that require a lot of running, jumping, and changing direction, for example, football or hockey, and affects muscles and tendons of the hip adductors. These muscles may be subjected to overuse or inadequate warm-up, sudden dynamic movements such as initiating a sprint, changing direction powerfully, or hitting the ground hard after a jump. They become overstretched or pulled resulting in tears of the muscle fibres. An adductor strain can also be acquired during heavy lifting using a poor technique; for example, if there is too much hip abduction and the lifting movement is not controlled then adductor strain might occur.

Presentation: The client can usually report an incident, likely during sport, when the injury occurred and remembers the onset of pain. Usually the pain is felt in the groin and inner thigh and is worse with adduction, especially resisted adduction. Walking and going up stairs will be painful. The severity of pain depends on how much damage has occurred, that is, on whether only a few fibres or a greater number are damaged, or whether there is partial/complete rupture. Bruising and swelling may be apparent.

Management: The client is usually advised to take simple pain relief and non-steroidal anti-inflammatories. They are also advised of "RICE": **R**est, **I**ce, **C**ompression, and **E**levation. They may be referred to physiotherapy for advice regarding prevention of re-injury and for an appropriate rehabilitation programme including strengthening and stretching exercises. If symptoms don't improve or rupture is suspected, referral to orthopaedics will be necessary and surgical management might be indicated.

Pilates programme for **groin strain or adductor strain**	Start by strengthening the core muscles without any pressure on the affected area. Introduce stretches and adductor strengthening exercises gradually. Work to address any imbalances (weaknesses) that could have contributed to the injury.
Contraindications/cautions	Don't exercise the affected area while pain and inflammation is present.

Recommended exercises	*Chapter*	*Exercise no.*	*Page no.*
• Prone gluteal squeeze	11	55	152
• Prone hamstring curls	11	56	152
• Pelvic tilts	10	35	131
• Adductor squeeze (soft ball)	8	3	92
• Leg work on reformer	8	9a, 9b	96, 98
• Assisted bridge on trapeze	8	12	103
• Knee drops	8	6	94
Progression			
• Ham string curls with extension	11	57	153
• Ham string curls with extension, abduction and adduction	11	58	154
• Leg work on reformer	8	9c, 9d	99, 100
• Bridge	8	11	102
• Clam	11	48	145
• Side lying leg work on reformer	11	52	149

6. Osteitis pubis

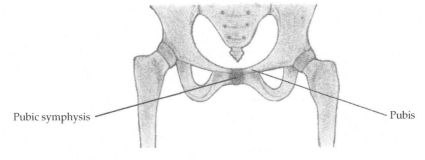

Pubic symphysis   Pubis

Figure 29. Pubic symphysis pain.

This is inflammation of the fibrocartilaginous pubic symphysis joint. The cause can be unclear but most commonly it occurs during pregnancy or with sports. During pregnancy ligaments become lax due to hormonal changes and the pubic symphysis joint becomes too mobile (often referred to as symphysis pubis dysfunction).

Osteitis pubis can also occur within sports where there are increased shearing forces at the joint, for example in football, ice skating, and dancing. Other causes include trauma, ankylosing spondylitis, and complications post urological surgery, but specialist physiotherapists are better placed to manage exercise and rehabilitation in these situations and can refer you to these when appropriate.

Presentation: The client will complain of pain in the pelvic region and might be acutely tender when the pubic bone is palpated. Adduction or abduction can result in discomfort as the muscles pull on the joint in either direction. Movement that causes unilateral shearing at the joint, such as going up and down stairs, or even just walking, may cause pain.

Management: Rest from the aggravating sporting activity is recommended. Simple pain relief and non-steroidal anti-inflammatories are indicated in the early stages. The client can be referred to physiotherapy maybe for exercise and rehabilitation.

As pain and inflammation subsides a Pilates programme of core stability, gentle stretching, and good postural alignment will be of benefit, and if a physiotherapist has been involved they can aid you with any particular areas to work on. This condition can be tricky to treat and can take a long time to resolve.

Pilates programme for **osteitis pubis**	Work to stabilise the pelvis concentrating on pelvic floor and deep abdominals. Strengthen gluteals and correct any posture faults. Keep a small ball or cushion between the knees where necessary and avoid opening the legs until pain has lessened.
Contraindications/cautions	Unilateral leg work, hip abduction.

Exercises recommended	Chapter	Exercise no.	Page no.
• Static abs (transversus and pelvic floor activation)	8	1, 2	91
• Pelvic tilts	10	35	131
• Prone gluteal squeeze	11	55	152
• Adductor squeeze	8	3	92
• Abdominal exercise with gym ball/roller	8	8	95
• Assisted bridge on trapeze	8	12	103
• Reformer leg work (add soft ball between thighs)	8	9a, 9b	96, 98
Progression			
• Small hip rolls	13	73	170
• Chest lifts	10	39	134
• Bridge	8	11	102
• Kneeling plank on reformer	8	13	104

7. Osteoarthritis of the hip and hip replacement

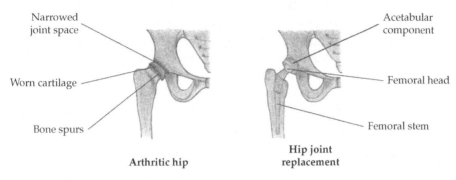

Figure 30. Arthritic Hip and Joint Replacement.

The hip is a synovial ball and socket joint where the head of the femur and the surface of the acetabulum meet. The articular surfaces are covered in hyaline cartilage that provides friction-free movement. As we get older our joints are subjected to a certain degree of wear and tear but normally they undergo a reparative process which is generally symptom-free. Sometimes, as in the case of osteoarthritis which affects synovial joints, the hyaline surface undergoes degenerative changes leading to the loss of smooth cartilage. This is followed by bone remodelling as you would expect but the new shape is not as it was before which can lead to smaller joint spaces, movement that is less smooth, and symptoms such as pain and stiffness. Surrounding structures are also affected with weakness of muscles and changes to ligaments and the capsule. Osteoarthritis is associated with increased age and is most commonly found in the hips, knees, hands, and feet, although other joints can be affected. Presenting age tends to be over forty-five but this is not always the case. Weight-bearing joints such as the hips and knees are more susceptible to "wear and tear" and osteoarthritis.

Presentation: Osteoarthritis of the hip causes pain in the hip area, the groin, and the back. The client may complain of a short period of joint stiffness in the morning and pain can be related to movement or weight-bearing and is often felt in more than one joint. As well as general decreased joint ROM, there may be also be fixed flexion of the hip. With osteoarthritis symptoms can differ from person to person and also between the different joints. The client can experience flare-up of symptoms which then settle down, and interestingly pain doesn't always correlate to the degree of joint changes seen on X-ray.

Management: Osteoarthritis does not necessarily worsen as you age and often lifestyle changes such as exercise and weight loss can be very effective in reducing symptoms. Your doctor can advise you on these areas and may also suggest pain relief and arrange a physiotherapy referral. Sometimes, if symptoms are very bad then further surgery, that is, a total or partial hip replacement maybe indicated (see below).

Hip replacement

If osteoarthritis leads to significant deterioration of the joint surfaces the surgeon may recommend a hip replacement (see Figure 30) which involves replacing the acetabulum with a single material cup (polyethylene, ceramic, or metal) and the head of the femur with a metal ball and stem fitted into the shaft of the femur (sometimes the head will be a different material to the stem). This is called a total hip replacement (THR). If only the head of the femur needs to be replaced this is called a hemi-arthroplasty. The other option that might be considered is resurfacing, where the surgeon removes and resurfaces the femoral head cartilage and place a prosthetic socket into the acetabulum. The way they fix the components for any of the hip operations discussed can either be cemented or cementless. With cementless fixation a material is used that allows natural bone growth around the prosthesis parts. It is important to know which type of hip operation the client has had in terms of:

i)   What parts have been replaced or resurfaced
ii) Whether it is cemented or cementless as this can affect early weight-bearing instructions
iii) Surgical approach (anterior, posterior, or lateral) as different muscles will potentially be moved or cut during surgery and weakened as a consequence, increasing the risk of dislocation.

Post-surgery advice regarding what movements should be avoided and early weight-bearing requirements have varied over the years as techniques change and advance. It is therefore very important that as instructors we work within our remit and follow very closely any post-operative advice from the surgeon and physiotherapist. You are unlikely to see these clients during the very early weeks when they are still under the care of the hospital or community physiotherapists.

Sometimes a hip replacement is offered after a hip fracture or for other types of arthritis such as rheumatoid arthritis, which we do not cover in this book; however, you can follow this management plan in close collaboration with the healthcare professionals.

Pilates programme for **osteoarthritis** **of the hip**	Work to strengthen the muscles around the hip joints particularly the glutei. Try to improve the range of movement (lateral and medial rotation) and stretch tight hip flexors. Include balance exercises and correct any posture faults.
Contraindications/ cautions	Avoid excessive weight-bearing exercises and reduce exercise if hip is inflamed.

Exercises recommended	Chapter	Exercise no.	Page no.
• Prone gluteal squeeze	11	55	152
• Hamstring curls	11	56	152
• Eyelash exercise	11	60	157
• Hip abductor exercise trapeze	11	51	148
• Side lying hip exercise	11	49	146
• Clam	11	48	145
• Reformer leg work	8	9a, 9b, 9d	96, 98, 100
• Standing iliopsoas stretch	15	86	188

Progression

• Hamstring exercise on trapeze	11	59	156
• Hip circles on reformer	11	54	150
• Assisted bridge on trapeze	8	12	103
• Hamstring curls with extension	11	57	153
• Standing hip strengthener on combo chair	11	61	157
• Iliopsoas stretches	15	86, 87, 88	188, 189, 190
• Quadriceps stretch	15	85	187

Pilates Programme for **hip replacement**	Work to strengthen the surrounding musculature (within the specified range of movement) particularly the gluteals and deep core muscles.
Contraindications/cautions	No hip flexion beyond 90 degrees. Do not allow leg to cross mid-line. No medial rotation.

Exercises recommended	*Chapter*	*Exercise no.*	*Page no.*
• Static abs (transversus and pelvic floor activation)	8	1, 2	91
• Pelvic tilts	10	35	131
• Leg slides	8	4	93
• Knee lifts	8	7	94
• Knee drops	8	6	94
• Prone gluteal squeeze	11	55	152
• Hamstring curls	11	56	152
• Eyelash exercise	11	60	157
• Glute med side lying with modification for THR	11	49	146
Progression			
• Clam with modification for THR	11	48	145
• Hamstring curls with extension	11	57	153
• Abdominal exercise with gym ball/roller	8	8	95
• Reformer leg work with modification for THR	8	9a, 9b, 9d	96, 98, 100
• Prancers	8	10	102
• Assisted bridge on trapeze	8	12	103
• Quadriceps stretch	15	83	183

CHAPTER SIX

Common conditions of the knee and lower leg

Relevant anatomy and movement
Conditions:

1. Ligament injuries
2. Meniscal tears
3. Arthritis of the knee and knee replacement
4. Achilles tendinopathy
5. Other conditions

Anatomy

The knee joint

The knee is a synovial condylar joint of the lower end of the femur and the upper end of the tibia. At the knee joint both the femur and tibia have expanded areas called condyles. Each bone has a medial and lateral condyle. Additional protrusions are found that provide extra areas of attachment for muscles and ligaments, these are the epicondyles on the medial and lateral femoral condyles, the adductor tubercle on the upper, medial surface of the tibial condyle, and the tibial tuberosity on the anterior part of the tibia. The kneecap, or patella, is a sesamoid bone embedded in the patella tendon and articulates with the patella surface of the femur. It is slightly triangular in shape with the apex at bottom and lies in a shallow groove, transmitting the force or the quadriceps muscle.

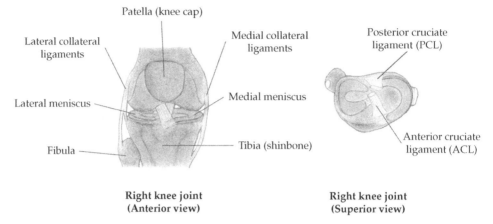

Right knee joint
(Anterior view)

Right knee joint
(Superior view)

Figure 31. Knee joint (anterior view) and menisci (view from above).

Muscle imbalance can alter the pull on the patella causing it to come out of its shallow femoral groove. The articular surfaces of the tibial and femoral condyles and the patella are covered in smooth hyaline cartilage. As with all synovial joints there is a joint capsule and this attaches to the margins of femoral and tibial condyles and also blends with the supra-patella tendon and patella ligament. Synovial membrane lines the fibrous capsule and secretes synovial fluid to lubricate the joint. The knee joint has several bursae which serve to reduce the amount of friction between tendons and bone.

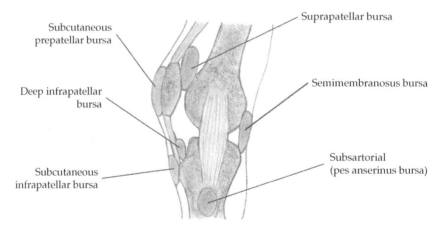

Figure 32. Bursae of the knee.

A number of ligaments (Figure 31) and tendons provide support to the joint: the supra-patella tendon which attaches the quadriceps muscle to the patella, and below this it becomes the patella ligament which attaches the patella to the tibial tuberosity. On the outside of the knee the extra-capsular lateral collateral ligament (LCL) runs from the epicondyle of the lateral femoral condyle to the head of the fibula and on the inside of the knee we can find the extra-capsular medial collateral ligament (MCL) running from the medial epicondyle of the femur to the medial tibial condyle. They reduce over-stretching of the joint in the frontal plane. Within the capsule, or intra-capsular, we have two ligaments that attach the inferior surface of the femur to the superior surface of the tibia. They are called the anterior and posterior cruciate ligaments (ACL and PCL) and cross over within the knee joint. These ligaments prevent excessive forward and backward glide of the femur on the tibia, that is, over-stretching in the sagittal plane and can be damaged during twisting injuries.

The cartilage or menisci (Figure 31) found on the medial and lateral joint surface of the tibia deepen the area with which the femoral condyles articulate.

Movements of the knee joint

The main movements of the knee joint are flexion and extension; however, there is an element of rotation when the knee is in full flexion which means that technically the knee is not a true hinge joint although it is often described as one.

Flexion: Hamstrings, with assistance from gastrocnemius and popliteus.

Extension: Quadriceps femoris.

Medial rotation (a small amount when the knee is in full flexion): Semimembranosus and semitendinosus.

Lateral rotation (a small amount when the knee is in full flexion): Biceps femoris.

The ankle and foot

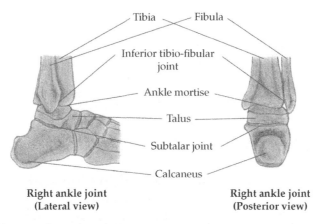

Tibia   Fibula

Inferior tibio-fibular joint

Ankle mortise

Talus

Subtalar joint

Calcaneus

Right ankle joint (Lateral view)   **Right ankle joint (Posterior view)**

Figure 33. Ankle joint (lateral and posterior views).

The ankle is a synovial saddle joint where the distal tibia and fibula articulate with the talus. Medially, the tibia terminates as the medial malleolus and laterally the fibula forms the lateral malleolus. A capsule is attached to the margins of the articular surfaces and extends from the malleoli to the talus. The lateral and medial ligaments provide stability of the ankle joint.

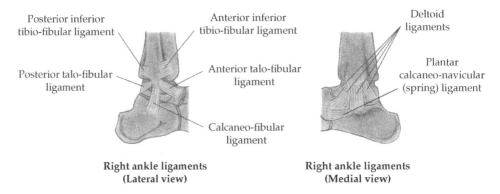

Figure 34. Ankle ligaments (lateral and medial views).

The foot can be split into three distinct parts: the hind foot, the mid foot, and the fore foot. The hind foot is the most posterior part and consists of the talus which articulates superiorly with the bones of the lower leg and the calcaneus, which sits below the talus. The articulation between these two bones is known as the subtalar joint.

The mid foot bones consist of the medial, middle, and lateral cuneiform bones which articulate with the fore foot, and the navicular and cuboid bones which articulate with the hind foot. The articulation between the fore foot bones and the mid foot bones is known as the mid foot joint. Finally, in the fore foot there are five metatarsal bones and distal to these are the phalanges.

Running almost the length of the sole of the foot we have the plantar fascia which is a fibrous sheath that attaches between the calcaneum (heel bone) and the bones at the base of the toes, covering the small muscles in the sole of the foot. During walking and running, as you "toe off", the plantar fascia becomes taut and helps the foot act as a lever to push off with force. It also helps to stabilise the medial arch of the foot.

Ankle and foot movements

Dorsiflexion and plantarflexion occur at the ankle joint and eversion and inversion occur at the subtalar joint. Below, the main muscles for each movement are named; however, there are other muscles that assist with each movement and the reader is advised to seek further information in more in-depth anatomy texts should they want to learn more. There are many small muscles of the foot, but it is not within the scope of this text to discuss these muscles here.

Dorsiflexion: Tibialis anterior.

Plantarflexion: Gastrocnemius and soleus.

Eversion: Peronei muscles.

Inversion: Tibialis anterior and tibialis posterior.

Conditions

1. Ligament injuries

Ligament injuries usually occur when a joint is suddenly moved outside its normal range resulting in over-stretching of the supporting ligament. If the mechanism of injury is forceful enough, a tear of the ligament may also result. The injury will be classified according to severity, from a mild sprain where only a few fibres are stretched or torn to complete rupture that will lead to joint instability. It is important to remember that as well as providing joint stability, ligaments also contain sensory receptors called proprioceptors that give the nervous system information about joint position. This in turn is important for limb function, mobility, and balance so must be taken into account when designing a rehabilitation programme; for example, using a balance board or BOSU ball can help to improve proprioception for ankle ligament injuries. Mild to moderate ligament injuries usually heal after around six weeks whereas more severe injuries can take much longer (a few months) to resolve.

Presentation: The client will complain of pain and tenderness around the affected joint (along the ligament line for the collateral ligaments), with a varying degree of swelling and bruising depending on the severity of the injury. There may be pain on weight-bearing and decreased function. If the injury is very bad and leads to significant rupture of the ligament and joint instability the joint may feel as if it is going to give way.

In respect of the knee, the MCL is most typically injured during sport such as football where there is a direct blow to the outside of the leg. The LCL is injured from a blow to the inside of the leg and injury can occur in games such as hockey where there are violent collisions. The ACL can be injured during non-contact twisting movement with sudden deceleration, for example, pivoting, landing, and jumping, or during a tackle from behind that pushes the tibia forwards on the femur. Often a loud pop is reported with immediate swelling due to bleeding within the joint and pain and giving way is experienced. Some 50–70% of ACL injuries are associated with injury of other structures such as the MCL and medial meniscus. PCL injuries are less common than ACL injuries and occur either from a hyperextension injury or a direct blow to the front of the tibia. The most common ankle ligament injury is an inversion sprain where the ligaments of the outside of the ankle are over-stretched and the client typically says that they "went over on their ankle".

Management: Initial management will consist of advice regarding pain relief, PRICE (protection, rest, ice, compression, and elevation), and how to return safely to activities and sports. Referral to physiotherapy may be indicated to further devise a safe and effective rehabilitation programme. If a more severe sprain or rupture is suspected with marked instability, or if recovery is slower than expected then the client should be referred to orthopaedics who will consider best management and whether surgery is indicated.

A good place to start is to work on the general strength and mobility of the leg, progressing the exercises as symptoms decrease. Include exercises that work on standing balance and joint proprioception, especially for ankle ligament injuries where balance board standing work is very helpful. For knee ligament injuries be aware that exercises involving a twisting or rotatory component of the knee may initially be uncomfortable and best avoided until a few weeks down the line, so to begin with you may just want to work in the sagittal plane. Always be guided by the medics and physiotherapist as to how you can best complement their management, especially if the client has had surgery. For example, with an ACL injury or surgical repair the professional advice may be to avoid open-chain quadriceps exercises at first as these can pull the tibia further forward on the femur.

Pilates programme for **knee ligament injuries**	Work to stabilise and mobilise the joint without weight-bearing initially then add more resistance as it progresses. Strengthen all of the surrounding muscles making sure to include exercises for vastus medialis.
Contraindications/cautions	Avoid rotation and generally use closed chain exercises (ACL).

Exercises recommended	*Chapter*	*Exercise no.*	*Page no.*
• Reformer leg work	8	9a, 9b	96, 98
• Prancers	8	10	102
• Knee exercise (with soft ball)	14	81	182
• Standing knee stretch on reformer	14	78	177
• Knee bend with TheraBand	14	79	178
• Quadriceps stretch	15	85	187
Progression			
• Reformer leg work	8	9c, 9d	99, 100
• Reformer single leg work	8	9e	101
• Leg work—wide position on reformer	14	82	182
• Knee/ankle mobility exercise seated on reformer	14	76	175
• Knee strengthening exercise seated on reformer	14	77	176

Pilates programme for **ankle ligament injuries**	Assess the strength and weaknesses of the whole limb and check for alignment issues. Work on stability and mobility of the ankle joint and only increase resistance as strength and mobility improve.
Contraindications/ cautions	Do not overwork or over-stretch injury (use graded exercises).

Exercises recommended	*Chapter*	*Exercise no.*	*Page no.*
• Reformer leg work with board	14	83	183
• Ankle exercise on combo chair	14	84	184
• Knee/ankle mobility exercise seated on reformer	14	76	175
• Prancers	8	10	102

2. Meniscal (cartilage) injuries of the knee

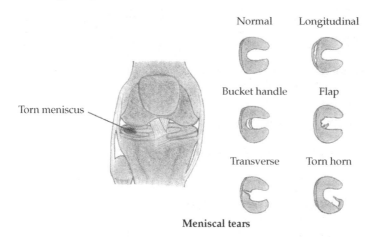

Figure 35. Meniscal injury.

A meniscal injury is usually traumatic in nature with an action that involves twisting or pivoting although sometimes the client is unable to recall a specific event. A tear can also be degenerative, seen more commonly in older clients.

Presentation: Pain is felt along the joint line and there will probably be some swelling and decreased ROM. If there is a tear that displaces into the joint, it can cause locking or catching, and the client may report being able to move the knee in a certain way so as to "unlock it".

Management: The aims are to initially reduce the swelling and pain and then get back to optimum function. Think of "PRICER": **P**rotect from further injury, **R**est and use crutches if necessary for the first couple of days after injury, **I**ce for 20 minutes at a time regularly throughout the day, **C**ompression with a bandage, splint, or brace, **E**levation and **R**ehabilitation which will involve a referral to physiotherapy for a suitable exercise programme if the symptoms are mild to moderate. If there is locking and a tear is suspected, or there is no improvement in symptoms after six to eight weeks of physiotherapy, then referral to an orthopaedic surgeon may be required. Surgery options include repair, partial meniscectomy (removal of part of the meniscus), or meniscal transplantation. The usefulness of surgery may differ depending on whether the injury is traumatic or degenerative.

Pilates programme for **meniscal injuries of the knee**	Work on strengthening, mobilising, and balance re-education. Check for any alignment issues and be mindful of the limitations of the knee. With age-related degenerative changes work on function and mobility and to minimise pain, whereas those with sports injuries will need to regain strength.
Contraindications/ cautions	Be guided by medical professionals.

Exercises recommended	Chapter	Exercise no.	Page no.
• Prone gluteal squeezes	11	55	152
• Prone hamstring curls	11	56	152
• Side lying hip exercise	11	49	146
• Hip abductor exercise	11	50	147
• Reformer leg work	8	9a, 9b	96, 98
• Reformer single leg work	8	9e	101
• Knee exercise (with soft ball)	14	81	182
• Remedial knee exercise	14	80	179
• Knee mobilising exercise seated on reformer	14	76	175
Progression			
• Knee strengthening exercise seated on reformer	14	77	176
• Standing knee stretch on reformer	14	78	177
• Hamstring exercise on trapeze	11	59	156

3. Arthritis of the knee and knee replacements

Osteoarthritis of the knee occurs due to degeneration of the articular cartilage of the joint. If we think back to the arthritis section of the pelvis and hip in Chapter Five, we will recall that the articular surfaces of synovial joints are covered in smooth hyaline cartilage that enables friction-free movement. As we age there can be some inevitable "wear and tear" and loss of this smooth cartilage. The reparative process is triggered but new bone shape may not be quite as smooth as it was before, leading to reduced joint space and changes to nearby structures such as muscles and ligaments.

Presentation: We will commonly see decreased ROM, pain, stiffness, instability, muscle weakness, and sometimes a fixed flexion at the knee.

Management: If symptoms are mild then general advice will include information about simple pain relief, regular exercise, addressing weight if this is increased, footwear recommendations, or appropriate walking aids or devices. If symptoms are

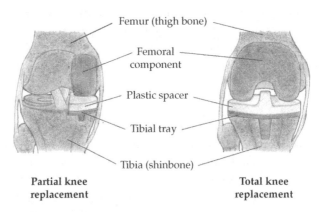

Partial knee
replacement

Total knee
replacement

Figure 36. Knee replacement.

more severe the client can be referred to physiotherapy for more specialist advice and carefully designed exercise programmes. If there is no improvement with these interventions, or if symptoms are very severe then surgery such as a total knee replacement (TKR) or partial knee replacement (PKR) might be considered. A PKR is sometimes called a uni-compartmental knee replacement because it only replaces the affected side of the knee, most frequently the medial compartment which is subjected to more wear and tear. This is less invasive than a TKR so there is a smaller risk of post-operative complications; however, the joint may develop further arthritis and require a TKR at a later date.

After a diagnosis of osteoarthritis by the doctor, depending on the severity of symptoms the client may or may not have been seen by the physiotherapist. If they have, then be guided by any physiotherapy advice and ask to see any exercises that they have been issued as these can be helpful when you a devising a Pilates programme. If they have come straight from the doctor having been advised to take up an appropriate exercise regime, your programme should include (as with many of the conditions that we have discussed) mobilising, strengthening, and balance re-education. If the client has had either type of knee replacement there are no contraindications to certain exercises as there are with a hip replacement, and exercise programmes should work on regaining strength, ROM, mobility, and balance. ROM can be quite decreased initially but we would hope to achieve and maintain at the very least, 90 degrees of knee flexion.

Pilates programme for **arthritis of the knee**	Work on strength and mobility of the surrounding musculature of the knee and correct any alignment issues that may be exacerbating the condition.
Contraindications/cautions	Do not overwork the joint particularly if inflamed.

Exercises recommended	Chapter	Exercise no.	Page no.
• Prone gluteal squeezes	11	55	152
• Prone hamstring curls	11	56	152
• Side lying hip exercise	11	49	146
• Side lying hip abductor exercise	11	50	147
• Reformer leg work	8	9a, 9b	96, 98
• Knee/ankle mobility exercise seated on reformer	14	76	175
• Knee strengthening exercise seated on reformer	14	77	176
• Remedial knee exercise	14	80	179
• Knee exercise (with soft ball)	14	81	182
• Prancers	8	10	102

Pilates programme for **knee replacements**	Work on a programme of strength and mobility in equal measure for knee replacements. It is important to regain ROM as soon as possible.
Contraindications/cautions	Do not overwork the joint.

Exercises recommended	Chapter	Exercise no.	Page no.
• Prone gluteal squeeze	11	55	152
• Prone hamstring curls	11	56	152
• Side lying hip exercise	11	49	146
• Hip abductor exercise	11	50	147
• Knee lifts	8	7	94
• Abdominal exercise with gym ball/roller	8	8	95
• Reformer leg work	8	9a, 9b	96, 98
• Knee/ankle mobility exercise seated on reformer	14	76	175
• Remedial knee exercise	14	80	179
• Knee exercise (with soft ball)	14	81	182
• Standing psoas stretch	15	86	188
Progression			
• Single leg work on reformer	8	9e	101
• Knee strengthening exercise seated on reformer	14	77	176
• Standing knee stretch on reformer	14	78	177
• Hamstring exercise on trapeze	11	59	156
• Quadriceps stretch standing	15	85	187

4. Achilles tendinopathy

The Achilles tendon (TA) of the gastrocnemius and soleus muscles in the calf attaches to the calcaneum or heel bone. It is the strongest tendon of the body, transmitting great forces during push-off when running and walking. Achilles tendinopathy occurs when the function of the tendon is compromised with resulting pain and swelling that affects the client's everyday function. Sometimes there can be complete rupture of the tendon.

Presentation: The client is usually active and will complain of an aching pain in the heel that can occasionally be sharp. They may experience swelling, stiffness after prolonged immobility such as sitting, and tenderness on palpation.

Management: Simple pain relief and rest from aggravating activities will be advised and gentle exercises can be resumed as pain allows. For acute injury ice or cold packs can be used. If there is no improvement within 7–10 days referral to physiotherapy is advised. If a rupture is suspected, then the client should visit Accident & Emergency that day.

A general Pilates programme should include strengthening of the leg muscles and graded stretches in order to gradually resume ROM. The area of tendinopathy has been researched fairly extensively over the last few years although best management still isn't clear. Treatment techniques and advice have changed, and no doubt will continue to do so. Eccentric muscle work has been shown to be beneficial and more recently it is believed that progressive and graded loading on the muscle and tendon (i.e. as symptoms improve) can be of benefit, moving through isometric (static) loading, isotonic loading, and finally plyometric (energy storage loading activities such as hopping or jumping). Be guided by the physiotherapist who will have designed a timely programme taking into account the amount and type of loading required. Try to correlate exercises with the physiotherapist's programme. If the client has been treated for a ruptured TA either conservatively or surgically, make sure you are aware of all medical or post-operative instructions.

Pilates programme for **Achilles tendinopathy**	Begin with non-weight bearing exercises and progress to eccentric exercises and gentle/gradual stretching of the tendon.
Contraindications/ cautions	Do not overstretch the tendon (particularly early in the rehabilitation programme).

Exercises recommended	*Chapter*	*Exercise no.*	*Page no.*
• Reformer leg work	8	9a, 9b	96, 98
• Foot work with board on reformer	14	83	183
• Prancers	8	10	102
Progression			
• Ankle exercise on combo chair	14	84	184
• Knee/ankle mobility exercise seated on reformer	14	76	175

5. Other conditions

There are many other disorders of the lower leg that you may come across in your Pilates practice, such as Osgood Schlatter's disease where there are multiple, small avulsion fractures of the tibial tuberosity. This condition is common in adolescents during the time of a growth spurt. Another condition that clients may present with is chondromalacia patella which is wear and tear of the inferior surface of the patella. This can be due to arthritis in older clients or if your client is younger it might be because the patella isn't running smoothly in the femoral groove of the femur due to muscle imbalance. This muscle imbalance around the patella can also lead to patello-femoral pain syndrome. Finally, it is worth mentioning plantar fasciitis which is a common condition associated with degeneration of the plantar fascia caused by repetitive microtears of the fascia. This leads to pain felt mostly in the heel and the doctor may make a referral to a podiatrist or physiotherapist. It is important that you research each condition that you come across: ongoing medical research means that management is always evolving. Be guided by any medical professionals that have been involved; for example, for Osgood Schlatter's the client may need to avoid open-chain quads exercises as they can pull further on the tibial tuberosity and in fact worsen the condition. But, as a general starting point you are looking to provide a comprehensive programme of strengthening, mobilising, and balance re-education exercises, many of which we have described for the conditions mentioned earlier in this chapter. Remember to think about what is going on regarding muscle balance and alignment in the whole leg and pelvis, not just at the affected joint.

CHAPTER SEVEN

Postural dysfunction

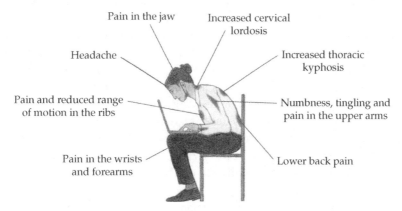

Figure 37. Poor seated posture.

Our posture is influenced by several factors including genetic make-up; a disease or medical condition such as arthritis, Parkinson's, or stroke; trauma such as a broken bone or habitual positions adopted in occupation, sport, or hobbies. Sometimes a postural dysfunction can be structural where the bones are incorrectly aligned from birth; for example, with a structural scoliosis which is a lateral curve of the spine (a curve in the frontal body plane). On the other hand, poor posture can be functional where our body has adapted to an occupation or activity; for example, sitting at a computer or carrying a baby on your hip. In these circumstances we might be able improve posture through exercise and change in habit or environment. Sometimes a client might have a functional scoliosis whereby a lateral curve of the spine has developed due to muscle imbalance that is secondary to something else. Examples of this might be after having a stroke, where one side of the spinal muscles can become weak leading to asymmetry; or after having a hip or knee replacement a slight leg length discrepancy alters the levels of the pelvis with a knock-on effect on the spine. Although it is not within the scope of this book to cover scoliosis in depth, we believe that Pilates can be of great benefit to clients with scoliosis depending on the severity of the curve and should be used in conjunction with the medical and healthcare professionals' input. We encourage instructors to have a look at the many books and courses available that address this topic and clients with a scoliosis should make sure they choose an instructor that has experience working within this area.

Another condition that can greatly affect posture is osteoporosis, a skeletal disorder where bone strength is compromised, predisposing the person to an increased risk of fracture. Bone is a live tissue that remodels itself according to need (a process known as bone turnover) but with osteoporosis this process is interrupted. Ideal bone density is achieved in the third decade of life for both men and women, with optimum flexibility and strength for normal function. After this, age-related loss occurs due to unequal rate of bone renewal. Women lose bone material more rapidly than men especially after the menopause when oestrogen levels fall. This is because oestrogen helps to protect against bone loss through its positive effect on bone remodelling. Men begin to lose bone mass at the same rate as women at around the age of sixty-five which is thought to be because of low levels of testosterone affecting bone mass density. Secondary osteoporosis can be associated with a number of medical conditions or where there is long-term use of drugs such as steroids: corticosteroids are thought to decrease the rate of bone remodelling. Risk factors for osteoporosis are heredity, femaleness, age, early meopause, hypogonadism, smoking, alcohol, decreased activity, and decreased body weight. As bone density diminishes the risk of fracture increases particularly at the vertebrae (especially the thoracic), the neck of the femur, and the wrist. Postural changes occur as a result of fractured thoracic vertebrae that collapse or change shape and we typically see a picture of thoracic kyphosis.

Bone density and internal structure can change with exercise and weight-bearing, making Pilates an ideal exercise regime for this condition. Not only does Pilates work to improve posture through realignment and core work, but it also offers a global strengthening and flexibility programme that moves through a variety of weight-bearing positions. However, it is imperative that instructors working with osteoporosis clients have experience and knowledge of this condition and its medical management which consists of current treatments and research, assessment techniques including scans, medication, and specialist advice. The programme often needs to be adapted to take into account the severity of the disease and the degree to which the bones are affected. The amount of weight-bearing you allow your client to do may have to be altered by changing position or offering adaptations; and movements that increase the risk of fracture must be avoided such as loaded spinal flexion or rotation.

When considering Pilates for postural dysfunction it is key to remember that each person has a body shape and posture unique to them and there is no "one size fits all". The way a client presents is dependent on a huge variety of factors that we have touched on briefly above. To begin with, presentation can be complex and overwhelming to analyse; however, a good starting point is to be familiar with the four main posture types that we discussed in Chapter One: lordotic, flat back, kyphotic, and sway back.

From there we have decided to consider lumbar lordosis and thoracic kyphosis in the context of two syndromes that we come across frequently in the studio: the lower crossed syndrome and the upper crossed syndrome. The lower crossed syndrome occurs in the lower part of the body in the lumbar spine and pelvic region where the lumbar spine demonstrates increased extension, or hyper-lordosis, and the upper crossed syndrome that is concerned with the upper part of the body has a main component of increased thoracic kyphosis or hyper-kyphosis.

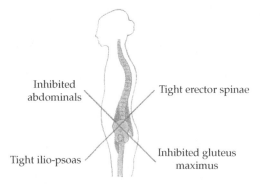

Figure 38. Lower crossed syndrome.

Figure 38 shows the lower crossed syndrome where we can see that the muscles around the lumbar spine and pelvis become lengthened or shortened with the characteristic patterns of weakness and tightness occurring in a diagonal cross between the anterior and posterior surfaces. Typically, we see overactivity and tightening of the lumbar spine extensors such as erector spinae and this corresponds anteriorly with tight hip flexors. The result is hyper-lordosis of the lumbar spine, increased anterior pelvic tilt and increased flexion at the hip and knee joints. Drawing an imaginary line between these tight muscles gives one line of the cross. The other line of the cross runs between the underactive and weak abdominal muscles anteriorly, and the gluteal muscles (maximus and medius) posteriorly. The thoracic spine may demonstrate a hyper-kyphosis as a way of compensating for the increased lumbar lordosis. Remember that there will be a knock-on effect throughout the joints up and down the body so look out for other consequences such as lateral lumbar shift, external hip rotation, and hyper-extension of the knee. These factors can all lead to further muscle imbalance and pain which will need to be taken into account when planning your programme.

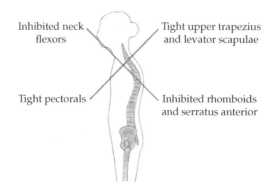

Inhibited neck flexors

Tight upper trapezius and levator scapulae

Tight pectorals

Inhibited rhomboids and serratus anterior

Figure 39. Upper crossed syndrome.

The upper crossed syndrome is demonstrated in Figure 39 where once again we see a diagonal pattern of muscle imbalance, this time in the upper part of the body. This is a common posture in today's world as more and more time is spent at desks and computers. The thoracic spine becomes hyper-kyphotic, the head and chin poke forward resulting in a lordosis or increased extension of the cervical spine, and the shoulders roll forwards. The muscles of the mid-back such as the middle and lower trapezius, rhomboids, and serratus anterior become long and weak and in correlation to that, the deep neck flexors at the front also become long and weak. In opposition, the posterior neck muscles such as the upper trapezius and levator scapula become tight, as do the pectoral muscles (major and minor) at the front.

Presentation: This will vary depending on the postural dysfunction, and a good knowledge of anatomy is essential in understanding why certain structures are tight or weak or why there is pain in various locations. To explain further: muscle imbalance produces joint dysfunction that results in ligament sprains and increased pressure on joints whether it is at the facet joints or SI joints, or more distally, through a knock-on effect, at the hip, knees, and ankles. Pain can be referred: for example, with the upper crossed syndrome clients may also complain of headaches that are cervicogenic in origin. Or, as the shoulders roll forwards with a hyper-kyphosis, the serratus anterior becomes long and weak, thus reducing glenohumeral stability and the pectoral muscles become tight, further altering the alignment of the glenoid fossa. This can then lead to a shoulder impingement.

Management: If the client has a specific condition such as osteoporosis or a congenital scoliosis, the medics may be involved to offer medication, investigations, or specialist input (for example surgery for a severe scoliosis). Physiotherapy is beneficial, offering manual techniques, exercise, and pain relief. As we say throughout this book, it is so important that you work within the guidance of the healthcare professionals.

Pilates management: Each posture will present itself differently to you, whether it is a lateral curve of a scoliosis or an increased kyphosis due to osteoporosis, or perhaps it is due to excessive computer work. With time you will become more confident with observation and analysis and recording of what you see. Your knowledge of associated pathology and common patterns of muscle imbalance will increase. To begin with try to note the areas or poor alignment and establish the areas of muscle imbalance. Try then to design a programme that can address these areas with the aim of improving posture and alleviating pain. The Pilates approach to managing postural dysfunction has to be holistic and flexible, remembering to think about the knock-on effect on joints or areas distal to the central problematic area. An instructor must be willing to customise the programme, taking into account the individual that they are working with, being mindful of cautions and contra-indications such as those mentioned for osteoporosis.

PART THREE

THE EXERCISES

To perform the exercises in this section properly, an understanding of Pilates is required. The breath, use of core, alignment, and mindfulness are important in executing them correctly. The breathing technique should be mastered first; then with an understanding of the neutral position of the spine and how the deep core muscles work to stabilise the pelvis, core strength will be obtained.

Pilates exercises are very subtle, and the slightest recruitment of the wrong muscles will override the exercise and negate the benefit. Only once this technique is mastered will the exercises have the required effect to help with rehabilitation.

For the purpose of this book and to avoid multiple repetition the *muscle focus* in each exercise will sometimes show the muscle groups only, rather than the individual muscles. Below is a table showing a summary of which muscles are used in each group in relation to joint movement or stabilisation.

Muscle groups	Primary muscles used	Secondary muscles used
Pelvic floor	Superficial muscles of the perineum, coccygeus, levator ani; pubococcygeus, puborectalis, iliococcygeus	Transversus abdominis
Deep abdominals	Pelvic floor, transversus, internal oblique	
Spinal flexors	Rectus abdominis, external oblique, internal oblique	Iliopsoas (sometimes)
Spinal extensors	Erector spinae	Semispinalis, interspinales, intertransversarii, rotatores, multifidus
Lateral flexors of the spine	Quadratus lumborum, external oblique and internal oblique (same side), erector spinae	Semispinalis (same side), intertransversarii, rotatores, multifidus (same side)
Spinal rotators	External oblique (opposite side), internal oblique (same side), erector spinae (same side)	Semispinalis (opposite side,) rotatores and multifidus (opposite side)
Main pelvic stabilisers	Pelvic floor, transversus abdominis, multifidus, gluteus medius	
Neck flexors	Longus capitis, rectus capitis anterior, sternocleidomastoid (SCM), longus colli, scalenes	
Neck extensors	Semispinalis capitis, splenius cervicis, longissimus capitis, splenius capitis, spinalis capitis, semispinalis cervicis	
Shoulder flexors	Anterior deltoid, pectoralis major (clavicular)	Coracobrachialis, biceps brachii

Muscle groups	Primary muscles used	Secondary muscles used
Shoulder extensors	Pectoralis major (sternal), latissimus dorsi, teres major	Posterior deltoid, triceps brachii
Shoulder abductors	Middle deltoid, supraspinatus	Anterior deltoid (>15 degrees), pectoralis major (clavicular >90 degrees), biceps brachii (when externally rotated)
Shoulder adductors	Pectoralis major, latissimus dorsi	Posterior deltoid, anterior deltoid, teres major, coracobrachialis, biceps brachii, triceps brachii
Shoulder external rotators	Infraspinatus, teres minor	Posterior deltoid, coracobrachialis (from internal rotation to neutral)
Shoulder internal rotators	Subscapularis, teres major	Anterior deltoid, pectoralis major, latissimus dorsi, coracobrachialis
Horizontal abductors	Posterior deltoid, infraspinatus, teres minor	Latissimus dorsi, teres major, middle deltoid (posterior fibres)
Horizontal adductors	Anterior deltoid, pectoralis major	Biceps brachii (short head), coracobrachialis
Scapula elevators	Upper trapezius, levator scapulae, rhomboids	
Scapula depressors	Lower trapezius, serratus anterior (lower fibres)	Pectoralis minor
Scapula protraction (abduction)	Serratus anterior	Pectoralis minor
Scapula retraction (adduction)	Trapezius, rhomboids	Levator scapulae
Main scapula stabilisers	Lower trapezius, serratus anterior, latissimus dorsi, levator scapulae, rhomboids	
Elbow flexors	Biceps brachii, brachialis	
Elbow extensors	Triceps brachii	
Hip flexors	Iliopsoas, rectus femoris, sartorius	Tensor fasciae latae, sartorius, gracilis, pectineus, adductor longus & brevis (early flexion)
Hip extensors	Gluteus maximus, hamstrings, biceps femoris, semitendinosus, semimembranosus	Adductor magnus (lower fibres)

(Continued)

Muscle groups	Primary muscles used	Secondary muscles used
Hip external rotators	Deep outward rotators, piriformis, gemellus superior, gemellus inferior, obturator internus, obturator externus, quadratus femoris	Sartorius, biceps femoris
Hip internal rotators	Gluteus medius (anterior fibres), gluteus minimus (anterior fibres)	Tensor fasciae latae, hamstrings, semitendinosus, semimembranosus
Hip adductors	Adductor longus, adductor brevis, adductor magnus, gracilis	Pectineus
Hip abductors	Gluteus medius, gluteus minimus	Tensor fasciae latae, iliopsoas, sartorius (upper ranges)
Knee flexors	Hamstrings, semitendinosus, semimembranosus, biceps femoris	Popliteus, gracilis, sartorius, gastrocnemius
Knee extensors	Quadriceps, rectus femoris, vastus medialis, vastus intermedius, vastus lateralis	Tensor fasciae latae (upper range)
Ankle/foot dorsi flexors	Tibialis anterior, extensor digitorum longus	Extensor hallucis longus
Ankle/foot plantar flexors	Gastrocnemius, soleus	Tibialis posterior, flexor hallucis longus

CHAPTER EIGHT

Pelvic stability

Pelvic stabilisation exercises are fundamental exercises designed to achieve strength and control from your core.

Imagine a cylindrical shaped structure inside your torso. The most superficial pelvic floor muscles are at the base of the cylinder, the deep transverse abdominals connecting with the multifidus are the deep wrap-around inner strength, the oblique abdominals are the outer wrap-around frame, and the diaphragm is at the top of the cylinder.

Once you have an understanding of this structure and it has been sufficiently strengthened, the limbs are able to move freely without unnecessarily moving the torso or causing undue stress to any part of the spine.

Breathing and deep core muscles

Breathing exercises

Breathing exercises or breathing control requires you to be very mindful of your breathing pattern. This breathing technique is used throughout the Pilates exercises. It is really important that we breathe properly as described below.

Place your hands gently on the sides of your torso at the bottom of your rib cage. Breathe in slowly through your nose and feel the air go down to the bottom of your ribs. You should expand gently to the sides of the lower ribcage and your tummy should rise a little but not puff out. Feel the gentle movement under your hands. Now breathe out through your mouth. The out-breath should be ideally longer than the in-breath. Feel your shoulders drop as the tension leaves them and your lateral tummy muscles draw in towards your spine.

A correct technique for the out-breath can stimulate better core stability as an important core muscle, transversus abdominis, is activated when you control your breath out. All this will have a positive effect on your postural control.

Neutral spine

Lie on your back with your knees bent and hip width apart. Put your thumbs and forefingers together to make a V and place the heel of the hand on your anterior superior iliac spine (ASIS—the bony parts of your pelvis) and the fingers pointing towards your pubic bone.

The pubic bone should be on the same horizontal plane as the ASIS and you should have a small curve in your spine. This is the natural curve of your spine so shouldn't be exaggerated or flattened.

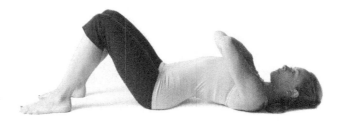

Figure 40. Anterior tilt.

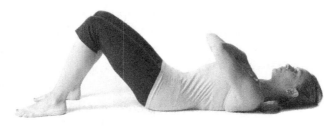

Figure 41. Posterior tilt.

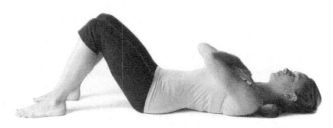

Figure 42. Neutral.

Pilates rest position and basic breathing

Muscle focus: diaphragm

Lie on your back with yours knees bent and hip width apart.

Feel that you have a natural curve in the spine (neutral spine) and that the two hip bones are on the same horizontal plane as your pubic bone.

Shoulders and ribcage should be relaxed with a feeling that your shoulder blades are sliding down your back with your arms down by your side.

> Place your hands on your tummy, breathe in through the nose, expanding the ribcage laterally (think of filling the sides of the ribcage with air but keep the abdominal muscles relaxed). Breathe out through the mouth holding the pelvis still.

1. Breathing technique using deep transversus (lateral) abdominis muscles

Benefits: *aids in achieving core strength and helps flattens the stomach*
Muscle focus: *transversus abdominis*

Lie on your back in the rest position (semi supine) as above.

> Breathe in through the nose, expanding the ribcage laterally.
> Breathe out through the mouth and imagine pulling the two hip bones towards each other making sure there is no movement in the pelvis. This is activating the deep lateral tummy muscles: transversus abdominis. Then add the pelvic floor activation as below.

2. Pelvic floor activation

Benefits: *helps to prevent stress incontinence and aids in achieving core strength*
Muscle focus: *superficial muscles of the perineum and levator ani: pubococcygeus, puborectalis and iliococcygeus, transversus abdominis*

Lie on your back in neutral spine with your knees bent and feet hip width apart.

> Visualise the muscles of the perineum, the superficial (lowest) muscles of the pelvic floor.
> As you exhale try to isolate this area and tighten the orifices (squeeze the openings) without engaging the buttocks.
> Continue with the above but also tighten the deeper internal sling of muscles (levator ani and coccygeus muscles) running from the coccyx at the

base of the spine towards the pubic bone and lift upwards through the torso. The transversus abdominis should also activate automatically as you do this.

By doing this you are activating the pelvic floor together with the transverse abdominals.

- Try to connect the bottom of the front of the ribcage with the pubic bone as well as pulling the two hip bones towards each other, so that all four points meet at the centre of a cross just by the tummy button
- You should feel that you are tightening (from back to front) and lifting the sling of muscles that support the organs within your pelvis
- Make sure there is no movement in the pelvis
- Do not allow the buttocks to activate
- Relax completely between each repetition.

3. Adductor squeeze

Benefits: *adductor strengthening with pelvic stabilisation*
Muscle focus: *hip adductors, pelvic stabilisers*

Lie on your back in neutral with the knees bent and a small Pilates soft ball or a cushion between them.
    Support the head with a small cushion if needed.

    Inhale to prepare.
    Exhale and gently, draw the knees together squeezing the ball.
    Feel the inner thigh muscles doing the work and activated from deep in the pelvis.

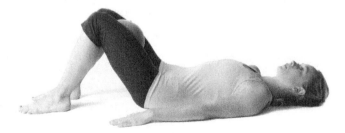

Figure 43

- Make sure you don't use the quads (thigh muscles) to push with the legs
- Feel the movement coming from the pelvic floor and drawing the knees together through the adductor muscles
- Keep the pelvis in neutral.

4. Leg slides

Benefits: *isolates the movement of the legs and improves hip flexor activation while stabilising the pelvis*
Muscle focus: *hip extensors, hip flexors, pelvic stabilisers*

Lie on your back in neutral spine with your knees bent and feet hip width apart.

Inhale to prepare.
Exhale and slide one foot along the mat as far as possible holding neutral.
Inhale and return the leg to the starting position.
Repeat with other leg.

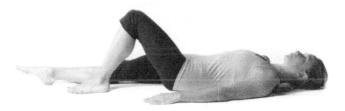

Figure 44

- Make sure your pelvis remains still while sliding the leg away and bringing it back to the starting position
- Use your deep abdominal muscles to activate the movement of the limbs.

5. Bug

Benefits: *isolates the movement of the limbs while stabilising the pelvis and the shoulder girdle*
Muscle focus: *shoulder flexors, shoulder extensors, hip extensors, hip flexors, pelvic stabilisers*

Lie on your back in neutral spine with your knees bent and feet hip width apart.

Inhale and take one arm up to ceiling.
Exhale and take the arm behind the head towards the floor as the opposite foot slides along the mat until the leg is fully stretched out.
Inhale and return the leg to the starting position and arm up to ceiling.

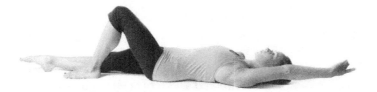

Figure 45

- Reach to the end of your finger tips but only take the arm as far as possible without losing neutral (lifting your ribcage or arching your back)
- Make sure your pelvis remains still when bringing the straight leg back to the starting position
- Use your deep abdominal muscles to activate the movement of the limbs
- Repeat on the opposite side.

6. Knee drops

Benefits: *mobilises the hip joints while stabilising the pelvis*
Muscle focus: *hip adductors, hip external rotators, pelvic stabilisers*

Lie on your back with your spine in neutral, knees bent and feet hip width apart. Support your head with a small cushion.

Inhale and allow one knee to open to the side, about 45 degrees.
Exhale and bring it back to the starting position.
Repeat 5 times with each leg.

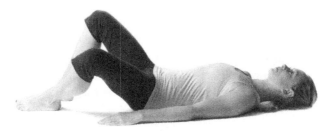

Figure 46

- Don't let the opposite hip lift as you open the knee
- Keep the abdominal muscles engaged
- Place the hands on the hip bones to help hold the pelvis still as you open the knee.

7. Knee lifts

Benefits: *improves hip flexor activation while stabilising the pelvis*
Muscle focus: *hip flexors, pelvic stabilisers*

Lie on your back with your spine in neutral, knees bent and feet hip width apart and support the head with a small cushion.

Inhale to prepare, exhale, draw in the deep abdominals and float the knee up to table top (where your hip and knee are at 90 degrees).
Inhale to lower it back to the starting position.
Exhale to raise the other leg to table top.

Breathe in to lower the leg.
Repeat, alternating the legs so you lift each leg 5 times.

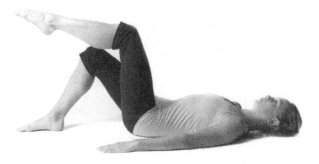

Figure 47

- Draw in gently with the deep abdominals to hold the spine in neutral and make sure the lower back does not arch or tilt when you are lifting or lowering the legs
- Keep the pelvis as still as possible with no shifting from one hip to the other as the knee lifts
- Move the legs from the hips, only without any movement in the pelvis at all
- Place your hands on your hips to steady the pelvis if needed.

8. Abdominal exercise with gym ball or roller

Benefits: *activates the deep abdominal muscles to work as control centre for the limbs*
Muscle focus: *hip flexors, pelvic stabilisers*

Begin lying on your back with both ankles on the ball, legs straight and together

Inhale to prepare.
Exhale as you draw in the deep abdominals and bend the knees—lifting them up to the ceiling as you are pulling the ball in towards your body.
Inhale as you straighten the legs back to the starting position.

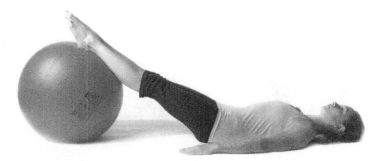

Figure 48

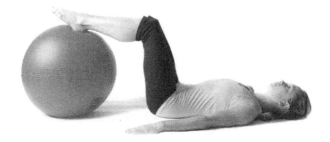

Figure 49

- Maintain neutral spine—do not allow pelvis to tilt posteriorly
- Think of the low abdominals drawing the knees in
- Add a little resistance as though the legs are being pulled in the opposite direction.

Modification of abdominal exercise with gym ball

For tight lumbar extensors/stenosis/spondylolisthesis etc.

- Do not maintain neutral spine—allow pelvis to tilt slightly posteriorly when the knees draw in towards the body.

9. Leg work,—reformer

A—Heels on bar

Benefits: *activates the deep abdominal muscles to work as the control centre for the limbs; strengthens quadriceps and hamstrings*
Muscle focus: *hip flexors, hamstrings, pelvic stabilisers*

Start lying semi supine on the carriage with your feet on the bar. Make sure you are in a neutral spine position and have a little space by the shoulder rests so as not to push against them and choose a spring weight that will allow you to hold this position.

Start with heels of feet on the bar in parallel, hip width apart and knees bent.

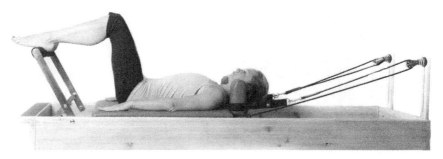

Figure 50

Inhale to prepare.

Exhale and holding neutral push back to full extension trying to squeeze the legs straight.

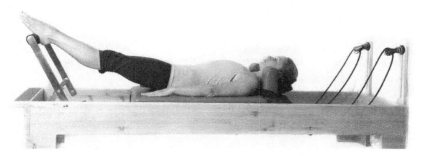

Figure 51

Inhale at top.

Exhale and try to initially bend the knees without moving the carriage, then keep lifting and bending them to the ceiling to return carriage back to the starting position.

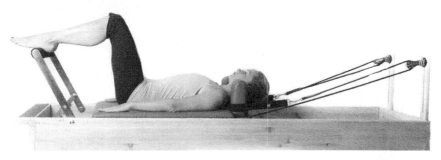

Figure 52

- Maintain neutral spine—do not allow pelvis to tilt posteriorly
- Weight should be evenly distributed across the heels
- Make sure the knees squeeze to full extension rather than a sudden jerk to straighten

Modification for hip or knee replacements

Move the carriage further away from the bar so that the legs do not go past 90 degrees when bent, or to an even less flexed position if needed.

Gradually move the carriage closer to the bar as the range of movement is able to be increase.

Modification for quadriceps strengthening

Add a heavier weight. Shoulders can touch the shoulder rests but make sure neutral spine is held.

Modification for more core strengthening

Take the springs lighter (blue only) and let the core do the work rather than the legs.

B—Heels lifted

Benefits: *activates the deep abdominal muscles to work as a control centre for the limbs; strengthens the quadriceps and hamstrings focusing particularly on the knees*
Muscle focus: *hip flexors, hamstrings, pelvic stabilisers*

Start with balls of feet on the bar in parallel and hip width apart, heels slightly raised, and knees bent.

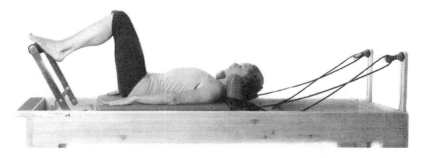

Figure 53

Inhale to prepare.
Exhale and holding neutral, push back to full extension keeping the heels slightly lifted.

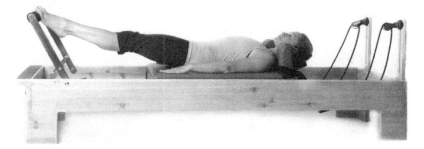

Figure 54

Inhale at top.
Exhale and bend the knees up to the ceiling drawing the carriage back to the starting position without moving the heels.

- Maintain pelvic-lumbar stabilisation throughout
- Keep heels slightly raised and don't let them drop or lift higher so as to work through the knee and hip joints only
- Weight should stay evenly distributed across toe joints.

C—V position

Benefits: *activates the deep abdominal muscles to work as the control centre for the limbs; strengthens the quadriceps, hamstrings, adductors, and deep external hip rotators*
Muscles focus: *hip flexors, hamstrings, deep external hip rotators, hip adductors, pelvic stabilisers*

Start with the balls of the feet on the bar in parallel hip width apart, heels slightly raised and knees bent. Externally rotate from the hips into a small V so that the heels are touching.

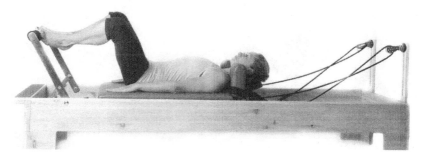

Figure 55

Inhale to prepare.
Exhale and holding neutral push back to full extension keeping the heels together and slightly lifted.

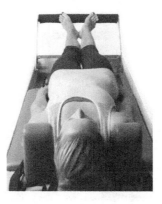

Figure 56

Inhale at top.
Exhale and bend the knees still in external rotation, and tracking over the feet draw the carriage back to the starting position without moving the heels.

- Maintain neutral spine throughout
- Pull up through the centre of your body as the legs straighten completely
- Don't over externally rotate from the hips
- Maintain alignment of feet, knees, and hip joints
- Try to keep the heels together throughout.

D—Wide position on heels

Benefits: activates the deep abdominal muscles to work as the control centre for the limbs; strengthens the quadriceps, hamstrings, adductors, and deep external rotators of the hips
Muscle focus: hip flexors, hamstrings, deep external hip rotators, hip adductors, pelvic stabilisers

Start with heels of the feet on the bar in a wide V position (edge of bar) and externally rotated from the hip joints.

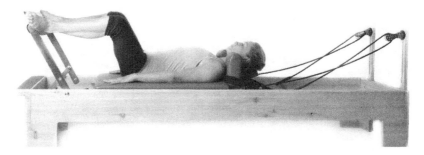

Figure 57

Inhale to prepare.
Exhale and holding neutral push back to full extension keeping the legs externally rotated.

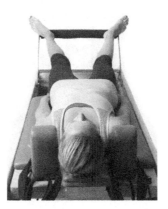

Figure 58

Inhale at top.
Exhale and bend the knees still in external rotation, and tracking over the feet draw the carriage back to the starting position without moving the heels.

- Maintain neutral spine throughout
- Pull up through the centre of your body as the legs straighten completely
- Don't over externally rotate from the hips
- Maintain alignment of feet, knees, and hip joints.

E—Single legs

Benefits: activates the deep abdominal muscles to work as the control centre for the limbs; strengthens quadriceps and hamstrings unilaterally
Muscle focus: hip flexors, hamstrings, hip adductors, pelvic stabilisers

Start with the ball of one foot on the bar in parallel, heel slightly raised, and knee bent.
Hold the other leg bent at table top or supported with the hand.

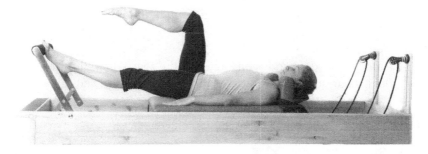

Figure 58a

Inhale to prepare.
Exhale and holding neutral push back to full extension trying to squeeze the leg straight.

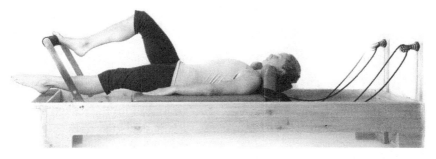

Figure 58b

Inhale at top.
Exhale and bend the knee up to the ceiling drawing the carriage back to the starting position without moving the heel.

Progression:

Place the extended leg under the bar to challenge pelvic stability.

- Maintain pelvic-lumbar stabilisation throughout
- Keep heel slightly raised and keep in that position (don't let it drop or lift higher) so as to work through the knee and hip joints only

- Weight should stay evenly distributed across the toe joints
- Connect the inner thigh of the extended leg with the opposite sitting bone to help keep the pelvis stabilised (progression only).

10. Prancers

Benefits: *stretches the gastrocnemius and soleus muscles and Achilles tendons*
Muscle focus: *hamstrings, quadriceps, gastrocnemius, soleus*

Start with toes on the bar in parallel, hip width apart and knees bent.

Inhale and push back to straighten legs.
Exhale, bend one knee and while keeping the toes where they are, lower the other heel under the bar to stretch the Achilles tendon and calf muscles.

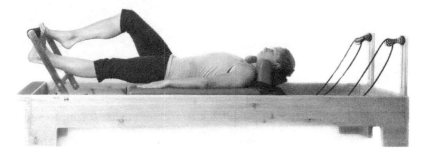

Figure 59

Inhale to straighten both legs then repeat on other leg.

- Keep the movement in the legs only, don't shift the pelvis
- Keep the stretch smooth and slow, don't bounce into the stretch
- Push the ball of the foot up into the bar as the heel goes underneath.

11. Bridge

Benefits: *strengthens the glutei and hamstrings; lengthens the hip flexors*
Muscle focus: *pelvic stabilisers, hip extensors, spinal extensors, hip flexors, shoulder extensors*

Lie on your back, semi supine with the feet hip width apart.
    Arms down by your side palms facing down.

Inhale through the nose expanding the ribcage laterally.
Exhale through the mouth drawing in with the deep abdominal muscles, push into the arms and the feet, and using the buttocks lift the pelvis straight off the floor into a shoulder bridge.

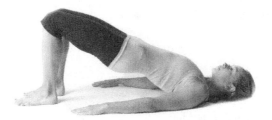

Figure 60

Inhale to lower.

- Co-contract the abdominal muscles and back muscles to lift the torso straight up into a shoulder bridge (no curling of the spine)
- Careful not to go up too high into the bridge causing the back to arch or the ribcage to flare
- Keep connecting the bottom of the ribcage to the pelvis through the abdominal muscles
- Make a good base for the bridge position with the arms and feet pushing into the floor.

12. Assisted bridge on trapeze

Benefits: *strengthens the glutei and hamstrings; lengthens the hip flexors*
Muscles focus: *pelvic stabilisers, hip extensors, spinal extensors, hip flexors, shoulder extensors*

Start lying on your back holding the curl-down bar above your head.

Place the trapeze bar approximately above your knees and then put your ankles into the strap with your legs straight and slightly externally rotated from the hip joints.

Inhale to prepare, exhale and lift your torso up into a bridge position while drawing the shoulder blades down and lowering the bar towards your legs.

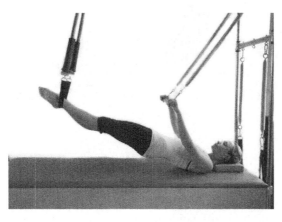

Figure 61

Inhale to return to the starting position.

- Make sure you use abdominals, buttocks, and inner thigh muscles to lift the torso
- Initiate the arm movement from the back: don't push with the arms or let the wrists flex
- Only use head rest if needed.

13. Kneeling plank on reformer

Benefits: *strengthens the shoulder girdle and hip extensors whilst activating the co-contraction of abdominals and back extensors to maintain a strong torso*
Muscles focus: *pelvic stabilisers, hip extensors, spinal extensors, scapula stabilisers, shoulder flexors*

Springs: As much resistance as necessary to hold position.
Kneel with hands on bar, shoulders over hands.
Make a straight line from shoulder to knee.

Inhale to prepare.
Exhale to move the carriage back, moving from the shoulder joints only and maintaining trunk stabilisation.
Inhale to return to start position.

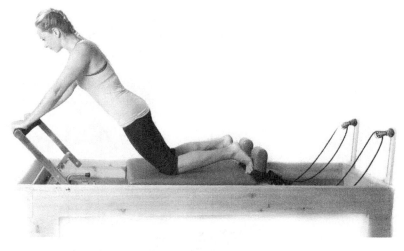

Figure 61a

- Keep hip extensors activated to maintain neutral pelvis
- Keep elbows soft and fingers and thumbs facing forward
- Keep head aligned with spine
- Maintain scapular stabilisation.

14. Tippy toes on soft ball

Benefits: *strengthens the abdominals and hip flexors without putting stress on the lumbar spine*
Muscle focus: *hip flexors, pelvic stabilisers*

Start in the rest position but place the soft ball under your sacrum making sure your back is not arched (pubic bone should be above ASIS) and arms at your side touching the floor.

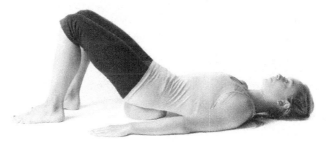

Figure 62

Take a few breaths in this position to stabilise the pelvis and get used to the feeling of being on the ball.
When ready:
Exhale and lift one leg, maintaining the balance of the pelvis.
Inhale to lower back down and repeat with the other leg.

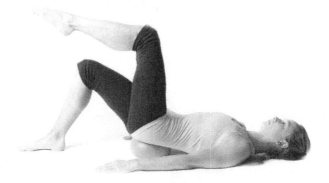

Figure 63

When ready:
Lift the heels and repeat as above but touching the floor with the toes only.

Progression:

Lift the arms to the ceiling and repeat as above.
Then change legs in the air just tipping the toes of one foot at a time to the floor.

- Make sure the movement comes from the hips only; the legs stay at the same bent angle throughout

- The further away you touch the toes to the floor the more demanding it is for the abdominals.

15. Butterfly on soft ball

Benefits: *relaxes and opens the lumbar facet joints*
Muscle focus: *hip abductors, hip adductors, pelvic stabilisers*

Start in the rest position but place the soft ball under your sacrum making sure your back is not arched (pubic bone should be above ASIS) and arms at your side touching the floor.

Take a few breaths in this position to stabilise the pelvis and get used to the feeling of being on the ball.
Lift one leg then the other to table top.

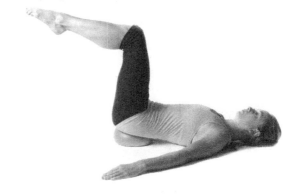

Figure 64

Inhale to prepare.
Exhale and open both legs to the side (like butterfly wings).
Inhale to close, then repeat.

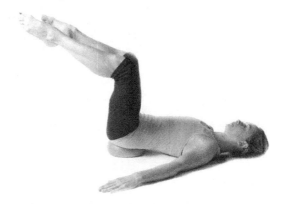

Figure 65

- Legs move from the hips only, they stay at 90 degrees throughout
- Make sure the lumbar spine doesn't go into anterior tilt.

CHAPTER NINE

The shoulder girdle

16. Dumb waiter

Benefits: *strengthens the rotator cuff muscles*
Muscle focus: *rotator cuff, scapular stabilisers, pelvic stabilisers*

Start seated on a chair or balance ball.
Make sure knees are aligned and level with hips (place a book under the feet if necessary to keep the knees at right angles with hips).
Start with arms bent and your elbows gently held into the waist. Your palms should be facing in with fingers long.

Inhale to prepare, exhale and rotate the arms to the side.
Inhale to return the arms to the starting position.
- Keep the elbows still—do not allow them to move behind body
- Don't lock the elbows into your waist
- Sit up tall with the abdominal muscles activated
- This exercise can also be done with palms facing down or upwards.

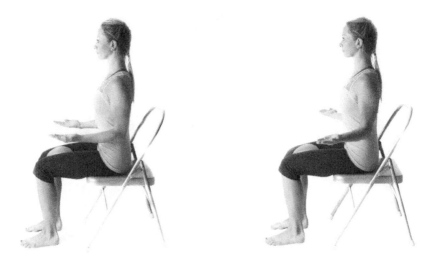

Figure 66   Figure 67

Dumb waiter progressions

16a. Use a TheraBand to add resistance.

16b. Perform seated on the reformer box or kneeling on the carriage.
Use a light spring to add resistance.
Hold the crossed stirrups in the hands with the palms facing upwards and the thumbs
pointing outwards (as though you are hitch hiking).

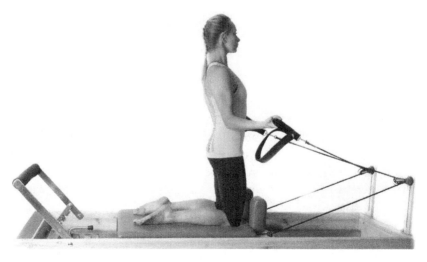

Figure 67a

- Keep the elbows still—do not allow them to move behind body
- Don't lock the elbows into your waist
- Lead with the thumbs
- Sit/kneel up tall with the abdominal muscles activated and hip flexors long
- Draw the bottom of the ribcage down to connect to the pelvis via the abdominals.

17. Seated plough

Benefits: strengthens the shoulder girdle and opens the chest
Muscle focus: scapula stabilisers, upper trapezius, pelvic stabilisers

Start seated on a chair or balance ball.
Make sure your knees are aligned and level with your hips (place a book under your feet if necessary to keep the knees at right angles with hips).
Have your arms down by the side (you can hold light weights if you wish too).

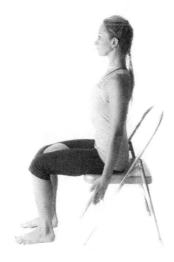

Figure 68

Inhale and shrug the shoulders up to the ears.

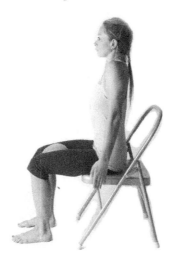

Figure 69

Exhale and lower them down while drawing in with the deep abdominal muscles and keeping the spine long.
Inhale and rotate the arms so that the palms face back.

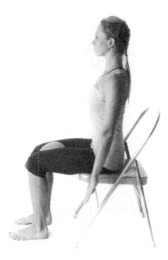

Figure 70

Exhale as you draw the shoulder blades down and move the arms slightly behind your torso initiating the movement from below the shoulder blades.

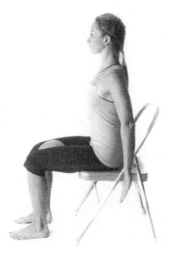

Figure 71

Inhale and return the arms to the starting position.

- Make sure that shoulders do not roll forward as arms move behind body
- Try not to let the ribcage flare
- Keep the abdominals pulled in and the torso still—only the arms should move
- Keep the back of the neck long
- Don't squeeze the shoulders back—it is a very gentle movement
- The arms should swing gently back and forth like a pendulum without any movement in the torso.

18. Seated plough on reformer box

Benefits: *strengthens the shoulder stabilisers and opens the chest*
Muscle focus: *scapula stabilisers, pelvic stabilisers*

1 blue spring
Start seated on the long box with knees on edge and feet resting over the head rest.
Hands in stirrups with thumb in and long fingers, palms facing back.

Inhale and sit tall with sitting bones pulling together.
Exhale as you draw the shoulder blades down and move the arms slightly behind your torso initiating the movement from below the shoulder blades.
Inhale and return the arms to the starting position.

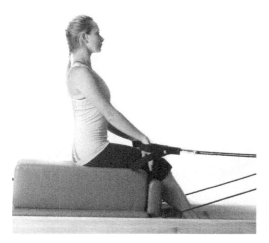

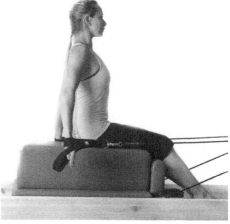

Figure 72   Figure 73

- Make sure that shoulders do not roll forward as arms move behind body
- Try not to let the ribcage flare
- Keep the abdominals pulled in and the torso still—only the arms should move
- Keep the back of the neck long
- Don't squeeze the shoulders back—it is a very gentle movement.

19. Arm lifts

Benefits: mobilises the shoulder flexors and extensors while stabilising the shoulder girdle and torso
Muscle focus: shoulder extensors, shoulder flexors, scapula stabilisers, pelvic stabilisers

Start semi supine holding a stick or TheraBand shoulder width apart.

Inhale to lift the stick up to the ceiling.
Exhale as you place the shoulder blades onto the floor, and take the arms back only as far as you can without the back of the ribs losing contact with the floor.

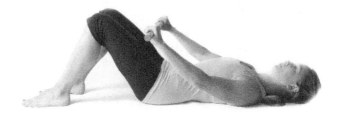

Figure 74

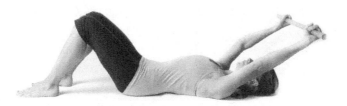

Figure 75

- Keep drawing the front of the ribcage down towards the pelvis as the arms go back
- Keep the abdominal muscles activated
- Keep the arms long but not locked.

20. Standing arm lift

Benefits: *strengthens the shoulder stabilisers while challenging the core*
Muscle focus: *shoulder flexors, shoulder extensors, scapula stabilisers, pelvic stabilisers*

Stand against a wall with legs bent so that your back is pressing into the wall.

Hold a stick or bolster cushion (just a little wider than shoulder width) in hands, palms facing inwards with arms long but soft.

Inhale to prepare.
Exhale, drawing in with the abdominals and lifting the stick up as far as possible without lifting the shoulders.

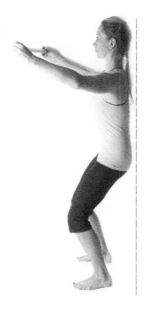

Figure 76

- Keep drawing the shoulder blades down as you lift with the arms
- You shouldn't go much higher than chest height
- Feel your core muscles connecting with your ribcage and keeping the shoulder blades from lifting with your arms.

21. Serratus cushion squeeze

Benefits: *strengthens serratus anterior unilaterally*
Muscle focus: *serratus anterior, lower trapezius*

Start seated holding a cushion or soft Pilates ball between one arm and ribcage with the arm bent at a right angle.

Inhale to prepare.
Exhale as you engage the abdominals, gently draw both shoulder blades down your back, and squeeze the cushion with your elbow feeling tension at the side of your ribcage.

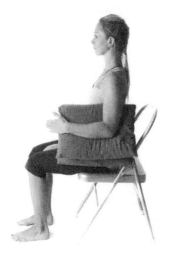 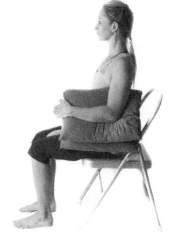

Figure 77   Figure 78

- Make sure that the shoulder doesn't lift up as you squeeze
- Try to feel the shoulder blade at the back of the torso connecting to the ribcage at the front
- Gently draw both shoulder blades down so as not to lean into working side.

22. Serratus exercise with TheraBand—kneeling

Benefits: *strengthens the serratus muscles with resistance while challenging the core*
Muscle focus: *serratus anterior, lower trapezius, pelvic stabilisers*

Kneel on the TheraBand with one hand holding the end at hip height, keeping the arm long but soft and palm facing inwards.

Inhale to prepare.
Exhale, engage abdominals, and draw down the shoulder blades as you lift the arm towards the opposite shoulder keeping the arm long.

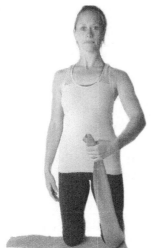

Figure 79

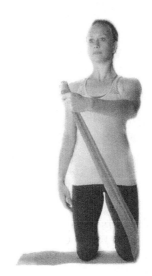

Figure 80

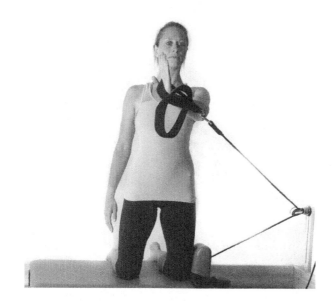

Figure 81

Progression: on reformer

Kneel sideways on the reformer carriage. Hold the stirrup (furthest behind) instead of the band.
Light spring only.

- Feel the connection between the shoulder blade and the front of the ribcage of the working side
- Keep the arm long but soften the elbow (don't lock it)
- Follow the line from hip to chest height at arm's length.

23. Deltoid arm lift

Benefits: *strengthens deltoid unilaterally*
Muscle focus: *middle deltoid, supraspinatus*

Start kneeling on a TheraBand and hold one end in your hand at the side of the body. Use only a light TheraBand to start with so that scapula stability is maintained.

Inhale to prepare.
Exhale to lift (abduct) the arm from the body against the resistance of the band while keeping the shoulder blade from lifting.

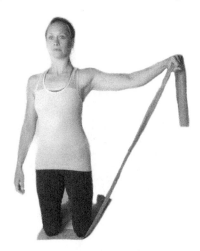

Figure 82

- Take care to stabilise the scapulae (draw shoulder blades down) as you lift the arm
- Only lift as high as scapula stability will allow.

Modification

This can be done seated on a chair with a very light hand weight.

24. Serratus exercise with TheraBand—supine

Benefits: *strengthens the serratus muscle with resistance while challenging the core*
Muscle focus: *serratus anterior, lower trapezius, elbow flexors, elbow extensors, shoulder external rotators, pelvic stabilisers*

Lie on your back in neutral spine with your knees bent and feet hip width apart.

> Lift one leg then the other and place a TheraBand around the feet holding each end in each hand with palms facing inwards, then straighten the arms and the knees to 45 degrees.

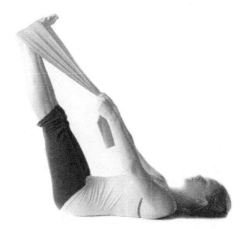

Figure 83

> Inhale to prepare.
> Exhale as you engage the abdominals, draw down the shoulder blades, and bend the knees, pushing the feet against the resistance of the band as you bend the elbows to right angles and rotate the palms towards you.

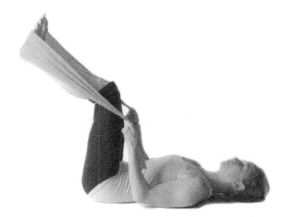

Figure 84

Inhale and return the arms and legs to the straight position.

- Use the TheraBand to create resistance in the arms by pushing the legs away from you as they bend
- Careful not to flex at the wrists.

25. Serratus exercise with springs—trapeze

Benefits: *strengthens the serratus muscles with resistance while challenging the core; can be done unilaterally*
Muscle focus: *serratus anterior, lower trapezius, elbow flexors, elbow extensors, shoulder external rotators, pelvic stabilisers*

Lie on your back in neutral spine with your knees bent and feet hip width apart holding the handles of 2 short yellow springs attached to the crossbar overhead (the bar should be roughly above the feet) with palms facing inwards.

Inhale to prepare.
Exhale as you engage the abdominals, draw down the shoulder blades, bend the elbows to right angles, and rotate the palms towards you against the resistance of the springs.
Inhale and return the arms to the straight position.

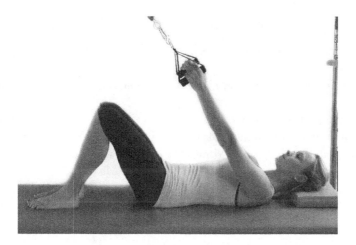

Figure 85

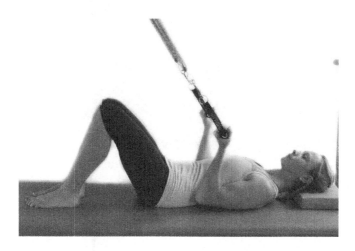

Figure 86

- Make sure you initiate the movement by drawing the shoulder blades down your back
- Only bend the elbows to 90 degrees
- Careful not to flex at the wrists
- Hold neutral throughout
- Move the bar further away if needed to increase the resistance of the springs.

Modification for single arm rehab

Start in same position but repeat using the rehabbing arm only, keeping the other arm holding the spring at length.

- Careful to still feel both shoulders stabilising even when using just one arm.

26. Shoulder rehab: arm slide and lift on bench

Benefits: *strengthens the serratus and lower trapezius muscles and shoulder flexors; can be done unilaterally*
Muscle focus: *serratus anterior, lower trapezius, pectoralis major (clavicular), anterior deltoid*

Sit sideways to a table or bench.
Place one arm palm down on the table surface with arm bent level with waist making sure that the shoulder can remain down (sit on books or blocks to lift your body up higher if necessary).

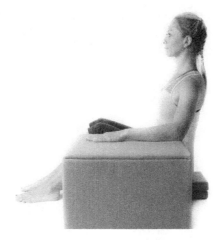

Figure 87

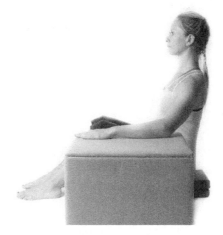

Figure 88

Inhale to prepare.
Exhale, engage abdominals, and draw down the shoulder blade as you slide your elbow along the surface—just a small distance (1 or 2 inches) without any rotation or movement in torso.

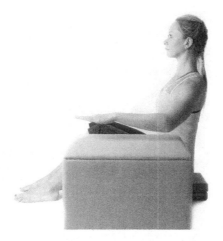

Figure 89

Inhale.
Exhale and try to lift arm very slightly, keeping it bent while still drawing down the shoulder blade.

- Do not let the shoulder blade lift as the arm lifts
- Feel that the lift of the arm comes from the back
- Keep the range of movement very small.

27. Cossack arms—supine

Benefits: *mobilises the shoulder joints*
Muscle focus: *shoulder extensors, shoulder flexors, horizontal abductors and adductors, pelvic stabilisers*

Lie on your back in neutral spine with your knees bent and feet hip width apart. With bent arms hold the opposite elbows up to the ceiling at right angles.

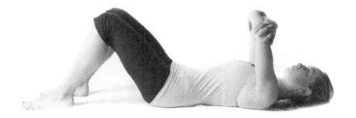

Figure 90

Inhale, then exhale and holding that position take the arms to one side feeling a stretch across the back of the shoulder.

Inhale back to the ceiling.
Exhale.
Repeat to other side.

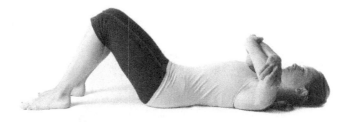

Figure 91

Progression

If able, once the movement is without discomfort, take arms in a circle; take to one side, then behind the head, then the other side, and finish back to ceiling breathing softly throughout. Repeat the circle in the other direction.

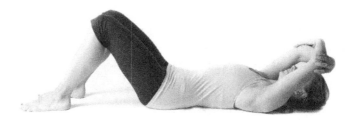

Figure 92

- Take care not to flare the ribcage when taking arms behind the head.

28. Arm circles

Benefits: *mobilises the shoulder joints while stabilising the torso*
Muscles focus: *shoulder flexors, shoulder extensors, shoulder adductors, scapula stabilisers, pelvic stabilisers*

Start in the rest position with your arms by your side and the palms facing in.

Inhale through the nose taking the arms up to the ceiling.

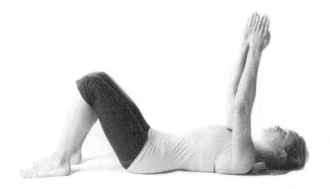

Figure 93

Exhale, placing the shoulder blades on the floor and stretch the arms behind your head, drawing the bottom of the ribcage down towards your hip bones.

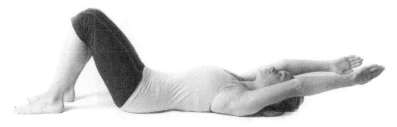

Figure 94

Inhale again, exhale as you draw your shoulder blades down, and leading with the little fingers circle the arms around the side and back to your hips.

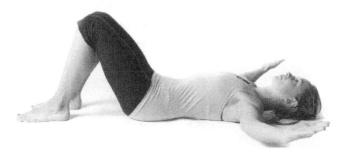

Figure 95

- As you stretch back go as far as you can without lifting the ribcage or arching the back

- While circling the arms back to the starting position relax the elbows slightly and draw the shoulder blades down away from the ears
- Imagine your arms are wings attached to your spine and controlled by the back muscles.

29. Shoulder mobilisation with TheraBand

Benefits: *strengthens the serratus and lower trapezius muscles and mobilises the shoulder flexors and rotators*
Muscle focus: *elbow flexors, elbow extensors, shoulder flexors, shoulder external rotators, scapula stabilisers, pelvic stabilisers*

Lie on your back in neutral spine with your knees bent and feet hip width apart. Take a TheraBand between both hands, shoulder width apart.

Inhale and lift the TheraBand up to the ceiling above the shoulders.

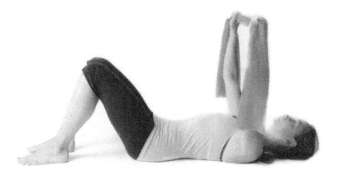

Figure 96

Exhale, engage the abdominals, and bend the elbows out to the side touching the mat.

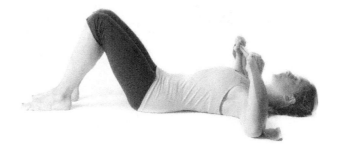

Figure 97

Inhale and rotate at the shoulders taking the band behind your head still with elbows bent.

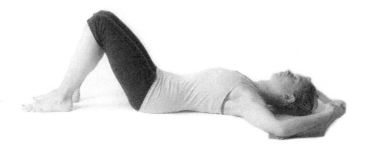

Figure 98

Exhale and try to straighten the arms along the floor keeping the shoulder blades drawn down and without flaring the ribcage.

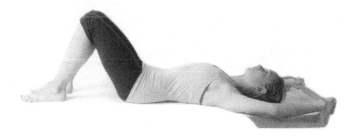

Figure 99

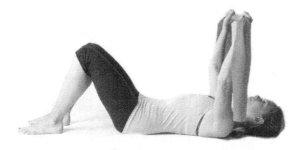

Figure 100

Inhale and lift the band back up to the ceiling.

- The spine should remain in neutral throughout
- Only straighten the arms as far as possible along the floor without flaring the ribcage or lifting the shoulders
- Keep the shoulder blades stabilised throughout.

30. Shoulder mobilisation with push through bar on trapeze

Benefits: *strengthens the serratus and lower trapezius muscles and mobilises the shoulder flexors and rotators*
Muscle focus: *elbow flexors, elbow extensors, shoulder flexors, shoulder external rotators, scapula stabilisers, pelvic stabilisers*

Lie on your back in neutral spine with your knees bent and feet hip width apart. Hold the push-through bar above the shoulders.

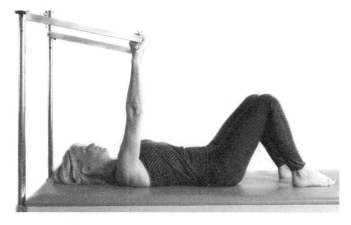

Figure 101

Inhale to pull the bar down towards forehead opening the elbows out to the side.

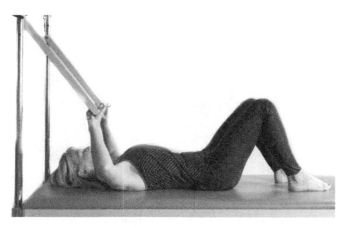

Figure 102

Exhale, draw in abdominals, and push the bar behind the head, straightening the arms as far as possible without flaring the ribcage.

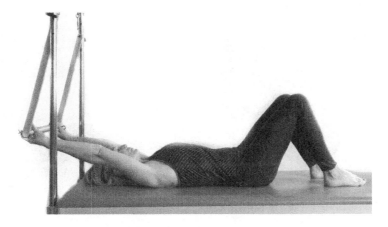

Figure 103

Inhale and bring the bar back to the forehead, elbows pointing outwards.
Exhale to straighten the arms back up to the ceiling.

- Do not lose neutral as you push the bar back
- The back of the ribcage must maintain contact with the bed even if the arms
  are unable to fully straighten.

Modification for shoulder impingement

- Keep elbows pointing forwards during exercise (do not open to side) and
  only push the bar back as far as possible without any discomfort.

31. Chin dips—seated

Benefits: *strengthens the neck flexors and lengthens the neck extensors*
Muscle focus: *neck flexors*

Sit on a chair and place your index fingers behind your ears and your thumbs under
your chin

Inhale to prepare, sitting up as tall and straight as possible.
Exhale and dip your chin down; pressing your chin into your thumbs,
draw your shoulders down your back; feel that you are lengthening the
spine from the bottom right up through the back of your neck.

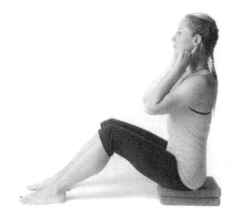 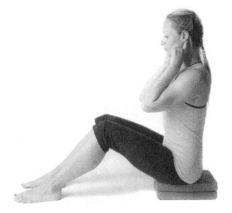

Figure 104   Figure 105

32. Chin dips on soft ball

Benefits: *strengthens the neck flexors and lengthens the neck extensors; can relieve tension in the neck and shoulders*
Muscle focus: *neck flexors*

Lie on your back in neutral spine with your knees bent or resting on a cushion. Place a soft Pilates ball under your head making sure your head is in a good position and your chin is not too high.

> Breathe into this position a few times feeling the neck muscles relax and the head start to feel heavy on the ball.

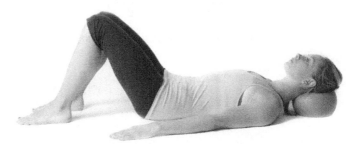

Figure 106

> Inhale to prepare.
> Exhale and dip the chin down towards your chest, imagining a soft peach under your chin which you mustn't squash.
>
> • Do not lift the head from the ball
> • Feel the lengthening through the back of the neck.

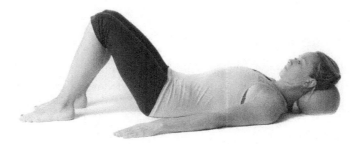

Figure 107

33. Head rolls on soft ball

Benefits: *relieves tension in neck and shoulders*

Lie on your back in neutral spine with your knees bent or resting on a cushion. Place a soft Pilates ball under your head making sure your head is in a good position and your chin is not too high.

> Breathe into this position a few times, feeling the neck muscles relax and the head start to feel heavy on the ball.
> Roll your head from side to side, keeping the soft peach (as above) under your chin.

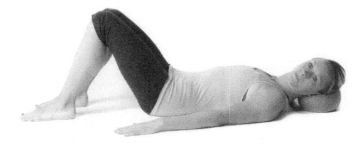

Figure 108

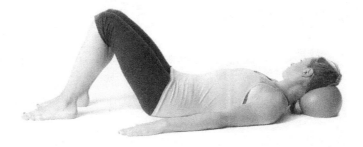

Figure 109

34. Shoulder joint release

Benefits: *relieves tension in ball and socket joint of shoulder*

Start by standing, leaning forward, and holding a support.
Allow the arm to hang down and make small circles from the shoulder joint.

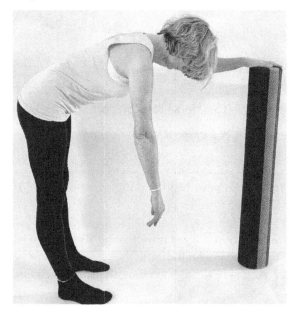

Figure 110

Alternative

Lie face down on a bed so that the shoulder is just off the edge; allow the arm to hang down and make small circles from the shoulder joint.

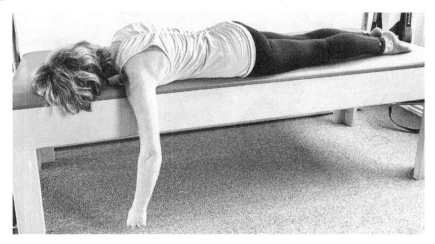

Figure 110a

CHAPTER TEN

Spinal flexion

Spinal flexion exercises are designed to strengthen the abdominal muscles while lengthening the spinal extensors (back muscles). In most cases the spinal flexors are working concentrically while the back extensors work eccentrically.

35. Pelvic tilts

Benefits: strengthens the pelvic floor and transversus muscles and mobilises the lumbar spine
Muscle focus: pelvic floor, transversus abdominis, spinal flexors

Lie on your back in neutral spine with your knees bent and feet hip width apart.
   Place your arms by your side with the palms facing down.

   Inhale, expanding the ribcage laterally.
   Exhale and while drawing in with the deep abdominal muscles, curl the pubic bone up just slightly off the floor.

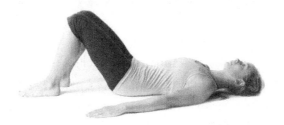

Figure 111

- The lower back should push into the floor as the pubic bone lifts
- Be careful not to shorten the torso
- Try to keep the distance between the ribcage and hip bones the same throughout
- Do not let the buttocks activate
- Imagine you are trying to curl the pubic bone towards your ribcage.

36. Small pelvic tilts on soft Pilates ball

Benefits: *strengthens the pelvic floor and transverse muscles and mobilises the lumbar spine*
Muscle focus: *pelvic floor, transversus abdominis, spinal flexors. Lengthening of lumbar extensors*

Lie on your back in neutral spine with your knees bent and feet hip width apart.
    Place a soft Pilates ball under your sacrum.

    Breathe in and out a few times to relax the muscles of the lumbar spine resting on the ball.
    Then perform some small pelvic tilts as above, keeping the lower back in contact with the ball (do not lift up).

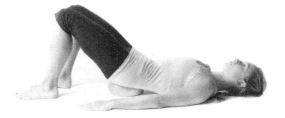

Figure 112

- Try to keep the distance between the ribcage and hip bones the same throughout
- Place your feet up on a chair with legs bent at right angles for more mobilisation of the spine
- Do not engage the buttocks
- Feel the lengthening of the lumbar spine as you curl the pubic bone towards your ribcage.

37. Larger pelvic tilts

Benefits: *strengthens the abdominals, hamstrings, and buttocks*
Muscle focus: *pelvic floor, transversus abdominis, spinal flexors, hip extensors*

Lie on your back in neutral spine with your knees bent and feet hip width apart.

Inhale, expanding the ribcage laterally.

Exhale, and while drawing up with the deep abdominal muscles, curl the pubic bone off the floor, then keep peeling the pubic bone higher one vertebrae at a time until you reach a bridge position.

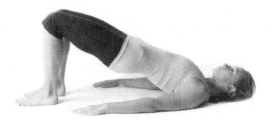

Figure 113

Take a breath in at the top.

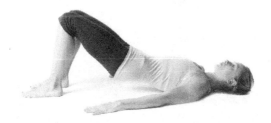

Figure 114

Breathe out while curling back down through the spine using the abdominal muscles to guide the pelvis down, articulating through the spine one vertebra at a time.

- Careful not to go up too high into the bridge causing the back to arch or the rib cage to flare
- The pubic bone leads on the way up but slows the pelvis (like a brake) on the way down
- Only engage the buttock muscles at the top of the tilt (bridge position).

38. Pelvic curls seated on reformer

Benefits: *strengthens the pelvic floor and transversus muscles while mobilising the lumbar spine*

Muscle focus: *pelvic floor, transversus abdominis, spinal flexors, and lengthening of lumbar extensors*

No springs—remove the spring bar if able.

Sit on a reformer carriage facing the foot bar with fingers touching the bar. Feet on the floor and knees at right angles to the hips (use blocks under feet if needed).

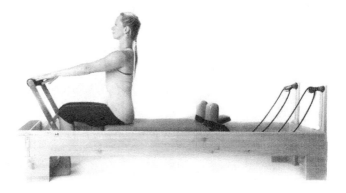

Figure 120

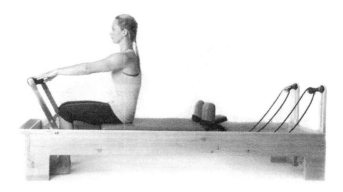

Figure 121

Inhale and sit up tall.
Exhale to lift up and in with the abdominals to create a pelvic curl drawing the carriage slightly forward while lengthening the lumbar spine.

- Try not to lose height while curling the spine
- Keep the distance between the ribcage and pelvis, don't let it shorten.

39. Chest lifts

Benefits: *strengthens the transversus and abdominals*
Muscle focus: *pelvic stabilisers, spinal flexors*

Lie on your back in neutral spine with your knees bent and feet hip width apart.
    Support your head with a small cushion.
    Place your hands behind your head with the fingers linked, thumbs running down behind your ears and elbows out to the side (just within your peripheral vision)

Inhale and drop the chin slightly towards the chest.

Exhale, draw in the deep abdominal muscles, and lift the upper body off the floor.

Inhale to return to the starting position.

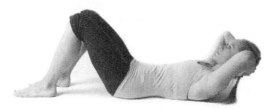

Figure 122

- Try not to let the pelvis move at all during the lift
- Think of lifting the chest rather than pulling the head up
- Imagine holding a soft peach under your chin that mustn't be squashed
- Try to maintain a stable pelvis—imagine it is strapped to the floor and only your upper body is able to move.

40. Oblique chest lifts

Benefits: *strengthens the transverse, rectus, and oblique abdominals*
Muscle focus: *pelvic stabilisers, spinal flexors, spinal rotators*

Lie on your back in neutral spine with your knees bent and feet hip width apart.
    Support your head with a small cushion.
    Place your hand behind your neck with left, and right arm resting across body.

    Inhale and drop the chin slightly towards the chest.
    Exhale, draw in the deep abdominal muscles, and lift the upper body off the floor while slightly rotating to the left and reaching the right arm towards the left knee.
    Inhale to return to the starting position.

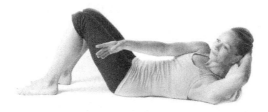

Figure 123

- Keep the reaching arm soft
- Think of rotating both shoulders as you lift: you are not rolling onto one

- Don't let the opposite hip lift up off the mat
- Try to maintain a stable pelvis—imagine it is strapped to the floor and only your upper body is able to move.

41. Curl down with TheraBand

Benefits: *strengthens the abdominals and lengthens the back extensor muscles*
Muscle focus: *transversus abdominis, spinal flexors*

Sit up straight with legs bent in front hip width apart and TheraBand around feet holding out to side with the arms long.

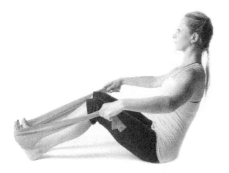
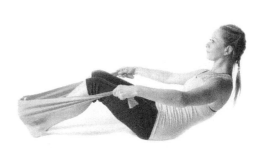

Figure 124   Figure 125

Inhale and hinge back slightly from hips.
Exhale and start to curl through the spine one vertebra at a time until you reach the bottom of the shoulder blades.
Inhale.
Exhale to curl back up to starting position.

- Keep the arms long and relaxed; do not use them to curl back up
- Start the curl down from the bottom of the spine rather than the shoulders
- Think of the bottom of the ribcage drawing down towards the sitting bones to activate the abdominals to sit you back up.

Progression

As the abdominals strengthen try to curl down further.

42. Curl down on trapeze

Benefits: *strengthens the abdominal muscles and lengthens the back extensors*
Muscle focus: *transversus abdominis, spinal flexors*

Use 2 long yellow springs plus curl-down bar (use the short yellow springs if little abdominal strength or difficulty flexing the spine).

Sit on trapeze, facing and holding the curl-down bar. Legs bent or resting on bolster or roller.

Inhale to hinge back slightly from the hips.

Exhale to start to curl down from the tail bone, through the spine one vertebra at a time.

Inhale when you have reached as far as you feel confident to go.

Exhale and curl back up, drawing the bottom of the ribcage towards the sitting bones.

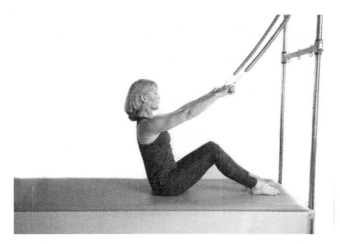

Figure 126

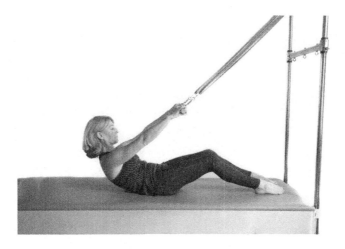

Figure 127

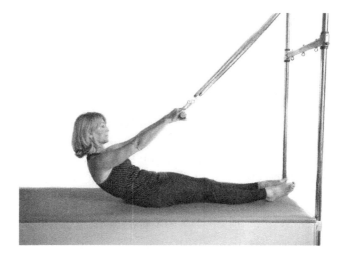

Figure 128

- Start the curl down from the bottom of the spine rather than the shoulders
- Try not to use the arms to help on the way back up.

Progression

Once you have mastered this and are pain–free, straighten the legs and go all the way down to lying flat before curling back up.

43. The cat

Benefits: *strengthens the deep abdominals and mobilises the back extensor muscles*
Muscle focus: *pelvic floor, transversus abdominis, spinal flexors, spinal extensors*

Start on all fours with the hips over knees and your shoulders over the hands.

Inhale to prepare, exhale as you draw the deep abdominal muscles towards your spine—drop the head so you are looking between the knees. Your tailbone should tuck under and draw down so that the back is arched like an angry cat.

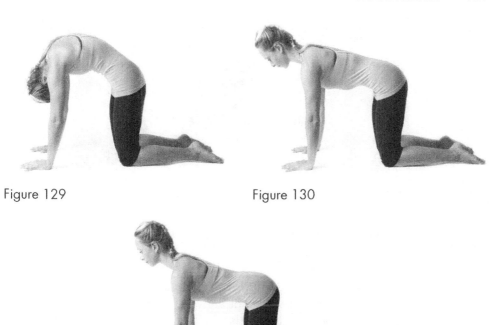

Figure 129   Figure 130

Figure 131

Inhale to come back to a flat back.
Exhale and arch the other way so that you are looking up and sticking your
bottom out—a happy cat!

- Make sure the movement starts with the drawing in of your abdominal muscles
- When the back extends into an arched position make sure the arch is through
  the thoracic and not just into the neck
- Place a rolled-up towel under the heels of the hands to take pressure off wrists
  if necessary.

44. The cat on reformer

No springs.

Benefits: *strengthens the deep abdominals and lengthens the back extensor muscles*
Muscle focus: *pelvic floor, transversus abdominis, spinal flexors; lengthening of erector spinae*

Kneel on the reformer with your hands on the frame under your shoulders and knees
up against the shoulder rests.

Inhale to prepare.

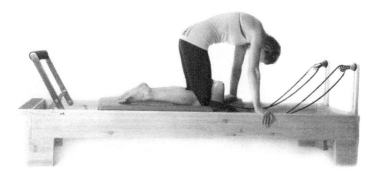

Figure 132

Exhale and draw the abdominals up towards the spine and curl into an angry cat position.
Inhale, stay in this position.
Then exhale, draw up again with the low abdominals, and push the knees into the shoulder rests and tuck them under your torso.
Repeat this each time on the out–breath.

- Careful not to move the torso
- It should be a very small movement of the legs only
- The movement should be initiated by the abdominal activation.

45. Mini curl up with push-through bar on trapeze

Benefits: strengthens the serratus and lower trapezius muscles and mobilises the shoulder flexors and rotators
Muscle focus: elbow flexors, elbow extensors, shoulder flexors, shoulder external rotators, scapula stabilisers, spinal flexors, pelvic stabilisers

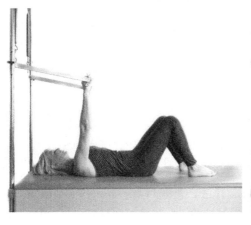

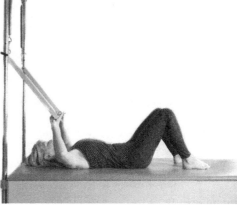

Figure 133   Figure 133a

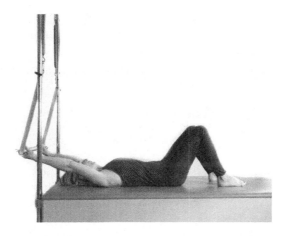

Figure 134

Lie on your back in neutral spine with your knees bent and feet hip width apart.
   Hold the push-through bar above the shoulders.

   Inhale to pull the bar down towards forehead opening the elbows out to
   the side.
   Exhale, draw in abdominals, and push the bar behind the head, straightening the arms as far as possible without flaring the ribcage.
   Inhale and bring the bar back to the forehead, elbows pointing outwards.

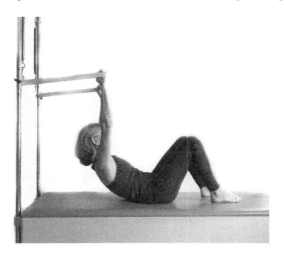

Figure 134a

   Exhale to straighten the arms back up to the ceiling, lift the head, and curl
   up into a chest lift.
   Lower back to starting position to repeat.

- Do not lose neutral as you push the bar back
- The back of the ribcage must maintain contact with the bed even if the arms are unable to fully straighten
- During curl-up only lift chest as far as possible without moving pelvis.

46. Lumbar stretch seated on reformer

Benefits: *lengthens the lumbar extensors and latissimus dorsi*

No springs—remove the spring bar if able.

Sit on a reformer carriage facing the foot bar with hands holding the bar. Feet on the floor and knees at right angles to the hips (use blocks under feet if needed).

Inhale and sit up tall.

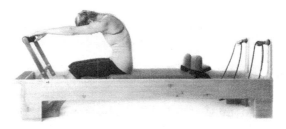

Figure 135

Exhale to Engage the abdominals drawing the tailbone slightly forward to curl the lumbar spine while pushing the carriage back and stretching the legs to create a stretch through the whole of the back.
Breathe into this position then return to the start.
Repeat a few times trying to gradually increase the stretch.

- Keep the shoulders from raising up too much towards the ears
- Try to feel the stretch though the whole of the back.

47. Lumbar stretch seated with gym ball

Benefits: *stretches the back extensors and latissimus dorsi*

Sit on a stool legs slightly apart with your hands on a large gym ball.

Inhale and sit up tall.
Exhale to engage the abdominals while pushing the ball forwards to create a stretch through the whole of the back.
Breathe into this position then return to the start.
Repeat a few times trying to gradually increase the stretch.

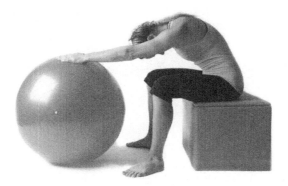

Figure 136

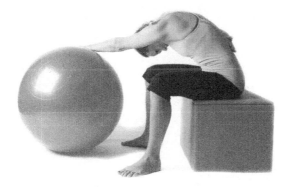

Figure 137

Modification

Place one hand behind your back and the other in the middle of the gym ball.

Repeat as above but push the ball to the diagonal to create a slight rotation in the torso and stretch one side of your back only.

CHAPTER ELEVEN

Hip rehabilitation

To maintain proper function and strengthen the hip joints it is important to balance the strength of the buttocks, hip flexors, hip extensors and adductors, as any tightness or weakness in these areas will have a detrimental effect on the function of the hips.

48. Clam (alternative to knee drops)

Benefits: strengthens the gluteus medius (posterior fibres) and deep external rotators of the hip, and mobilises the hip joint
Muscle focus: posterior fibres of gluteus medius, deep external hip rotators, pelvic stabilisers

Lie on your side (preferably against a wall).

Support the head with a cushion and place a rolled-up towel or your hand under your waist to support the gentle curve of your waist.

Have the hips and knees bent at about a 60-degree angle with the feet in line with the spine.

> Inhale to prepare, exhale and draw in with the deep abdominal muscles, and lift the top knee towards the ceiling keeping the feet together and without moving the pelvis.
> Exhale and place the knee back to starting position.

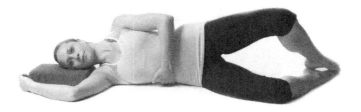

Figure 138

- Try not to sink into the towel with your waist: think of lifting away from the towel with the abdominal muscles and this will help to hold the hips still
- Try not to rock the top hip backwards
- Initiate the opening hinge movement from the deep buttock muscles.

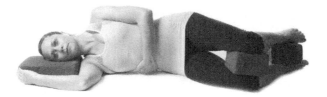

Figure 139

Modification for hip replacement

Perform the exercise as above but place a cushion between the knees and one between the ankles (so that the top leg is on the same level as the hip).

49. Side lying hip exercise

Benefits: *isolates and strengthens the gluteus medius muscle*
Muscle focus: *hip abductors, pelvic stabilisers*

Lie on your side (preferably against a wall).
    Support the head with a cushion and make sure hips are aligned keeping a slight lift under the waist.
    Bend the bottom leg; keep the top leg straight with the foot relaxed.

    Inhale to prepare, exhale, draw in with the deep abdominal muscles, and lift the top leg as high as possible towards the ceiling without moving the pelvis (you shouldn't be able to go much higher than hip height).
    Inhale to lower the leg.

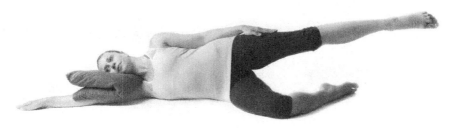

Figure 140

- Make sure the knee faces forward—don't let it turn up to the ceiling as you lift the leg
- You should feel the gluteus medius engage on the side of the buttocks, working to hold the pelvis stable as you lift the leg.

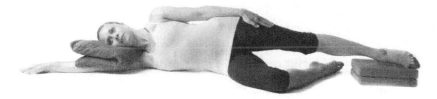

Figure 141

Modification for hip replacements

Perform the exercise as above but place some blocks under the working foot to reduce the range of movement.

50. Hip abductor exercise

Benefits: *strengthens all of the hip abductor muscles*
Muscle focus: *hip abductors, pelvic stabilisers*

Lie on your side (preferably against a wall).

Support the head with a cushion and make sure hips are aligned keeping a slight lift under the waist.

Bend the bottom leg; keep the top leg straight with the foot flexed (toes pulled forward) and foot resting on blocks (if needed).

Inhale to prepare, exhale, draw in with the deep tummy muscles, and lift the top leg as high as possible towards the ceiling without moving the pelvis (you shouldn't be able to go much higher than hip height).
Inhale to lower the leg.
Exhale and repeat again.

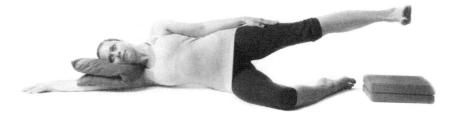

Figure 142

- Make sure the knee faces forward—don't let the hip externally rotate as you lift the leg
- Try to imagine that you are pushing up against water as you lift the leg.

Progression
- Without using the blocks hover the leg just above the floor without resting during the inhale phase.

51. Hip abductor exercise on trapeze

Benefits: *gently strengthens the hip abductors without lifting against gravity*
Muscle focus: *hip abductors, pelvic stabilisers*

Start lying in the rest position and place one foot in a stirrup attached to a long purple spring which is hooked to the middle crossbar almost directly above the foot with the leg straight.

Inhale to prepare.
Exhale, draw in with the deep tummy muscles, and take the stirrup leg down towards the bed against the resistance of the spring and then directly out to the side as far as possible without moving the pelvis.
Inhale and take the leg back to the starting position.
Exhale and repeat again.

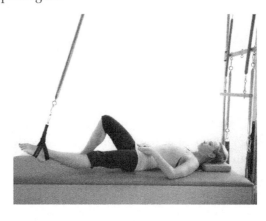

Figure 143

- Make sure the knee faces upwards throughout—don't let it turn out as you take the leg to the side.

52. Side lying leg work on reformer

Benefits: works to strengthen the hip and knee flexors while keeping hip/knee alignment
Muscle focus: hip flexors, hip extensors, knee extensors, ankle plantar flexors, ankle dorsi flexors, pelvic stabilisers

Springs: light to medium.

Start lying on your side on the carriage with pillow under your head and top foot on the foot bar with the leg bent and heel slightly lifted.
  Place one arm around shoulder rest and the other under gap at waist.

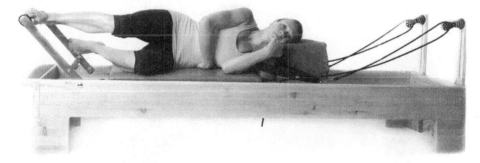

Figure 144

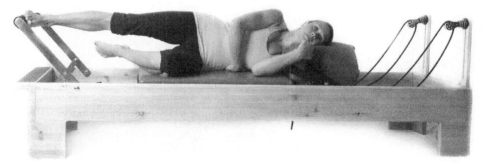

Figure 145

Exhale to extend leg fully, lowering heel.
Inhale to lift heel.
Lower heel.
Exhale as you return slowly to flexed position keeping the knee at same level as the hip and allowing the heel to lift as necessary.

- Maintain neutral spine—do not drop into waist
- Maintain hip/knee alignment throughout
- Lower and lift heel as necessary depending on the length of the Achilles tendon.

53. Hip circles with TheraBand

Benefits: *mobilises ball and socket joint of the hip*
Muscle focus: *hip abductors, hip adductors, pelvic stabilisers*

Lie supine on floor, lift one leg and place a TheraBand around the foot, holding with hands.

Inhale to prepare and straighten the leg to a comfortable position for the hamstrings.
Exhale and, holding the pelvis still, circle the leg around moving from the hip joint only.

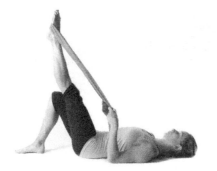

Figure 146

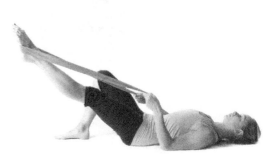

Figure 147

- Keep the toes pointed up to the ceiling
- Bend the other leg up if uncomfortable on the lower back or for very tight hamstrings
- Hold the torso still and feel that you are mobilising the hip joint only.

54. Hip circles on reformer

Benefits: *mobilises the hip joints while stabilising the pelvis*
Muscle focus: *hip abductors, hip adductors, pelvic stabilisers*

Springs: 1 blue and 1 red or 2 red springs.

Lie with feet in stirrups and legs straight at a 45-degree angle.

Holding the pelvis still, circle the legs down and around in a movement from the hip joints only.

Repeat up to 10 times, then change direction, this time going up first and then back down and around.

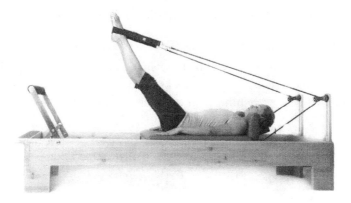

Figure 148

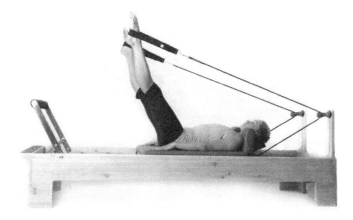

Figure 149

- Keep the breathing relaxed and rhythmical throughout the exercise
- Keep the legs parallel (with the knees facing up to the ceiling) throughout the circle
- Be careful not to go too high or too low with the leg: keep the circle fairly small around the 45-degree angle
- Try to lead with the toes and reach out with long legs but without locking the knees
- Hold the torso still and feel that you are mobilising the hip joints only.

Progression: To increase hip mobility hip circles can also be done in external rotation.

55. Prone gluteal squeeze

Benefits: *isolates and strengthens the glutei*
Muscle focus: *gluteus medius and minimus, lower fibres of gluteus maximus, pelvic stabilisers*

Lie face down with legs straight, bend your elbows, and rest your forehead on your hands.

> Inhale to prepare, exhale as you draw in gently with the deep abdominal muscles, and squeeze your buttocks from the outside inwards towards your spine while lengthening your tailbone towards your ankles.

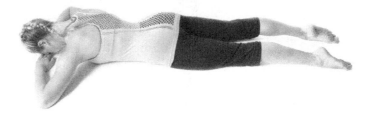

Figure 150

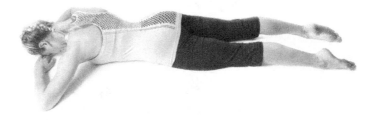

Figure 151

- Place a pillow under your tummy if you feel discomfort in your lower back
- Try to hold the spine in neutral in this position.

56. Hamstring curls

Benefits: *strengthens the glutei and hamstrings*
Muscle focus: *glutei, hamstrings, pelvic stabilisers*

Lie face down with legs straight, bend your elbows, and rest your forehead on your hands.

> Inhale to prepare.
> Exhale as you draw in gently with the deep abdominal muscles, squeeze your buttocks as above, and bend one leg to 90 degrees keeping the knee on the floor.

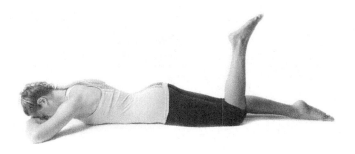

Figure 152

- Make sure the heel of the working leg tracks in line with the buttock
- Try to hold the spine in neutral in this position—don't let the back arch
- Feel the back of the leg (hamstrings) working in unison with the lower part of your buttock
- Place a pillow under your tummy if you feel discomfort in your lower back.

57. Hamstring curls with extension

Benefits: *strengthens the glutei and hamstrings; lengthens the hip flexors*
Muscle focus: *glutei, hamstrings, pelvic stabilisers*

Lie face down with legs straight, bend your elbows, and rest your forehead on your hands.

Inhale to prepare.
Exhale as you draw in gently with the deep abdominal muscles, squeeze your buttocks as above, and bend one leg to 90 degrees keeping the knee on the floor.
Inhale and lift the knee slightly off the floor without any anterior tilt (arching of the back).

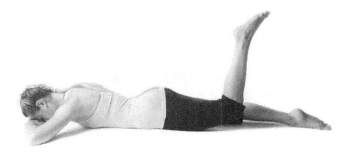

Figure 153

Exhale and extend the leg to straight at the same level as the knee (don't lift higher).
Inhale to lower.

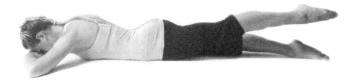

Figure 154

Repeat on other leg.

- Make sure the heel of the working leg tracks in line with the buttock
- Try to hold the spine in neutral in this position—don't let the back arch
- Feel the back of the leg (hamstrings) working in unison with the lower part of your buttock
- Place a pillow under your tummy if you feel discomfort in your lower back.

58. Hamstring curls with extension, abduction, and adduction

Benefits: *strengthens the glutei, hamstrings, adductor and abductors of the hips; lengthens the hip flexors*
Muscle focus: *glutei, hamstrings, hip abductors and adductors, pelvic stabilisers*

Lie face down with legs straight, bend your elbows, and rest your forehead on your hands.

Inhale to prepare.
Exhale as you draw in gently with the deep abdominal muscles, squeeze your buttocks as above, and bend one leg to 90 degrees keeping the knee on the floor.
Inhale and lift the knee slightly off the floor without any anterior tilt (arching of the back).
Exhale and extend the leg to straight at the same level as the knee (don't lift higher) and point the foot.

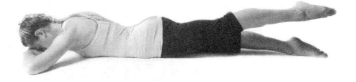

Figure 155

Inhale to externally rotate from the hip (turn out) and flex the foot.

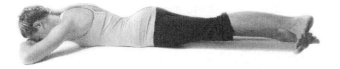

Figure 156

Exhale to take the leg out to the side.

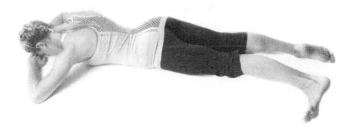

Figure 157

Inhale to bring back to centre.

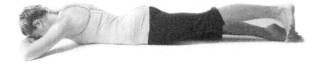

Figure 158

Exhale to point the foot and rotate the leg back to parallel.

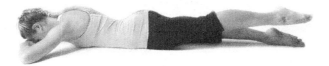

Figure 159

Inhale to lower.
- Make sure the heel of the working leg tracks in line with the buttock
- Try to hold the spine in neutral in this position—don't let the back arch
- Feel the back of the leg (hamstrings) working in unison with the lower part of your buttock
- Move the leg from the top only as you abduct and adduct, keeping it straight throughout
- Place a pillow under your tummy if you feel discomfort in your lower back.

59. Hamstring exercise on trapeze

Benefits: *strengthens and stretches the hamstrings using resistance*
Muscle focus: *hamstrings, pelvic stabilisers*

Springs: Long purple attached to middle hook (choose height to suit resistance and ability).

Start lying semi supine with one foot in a stirrup attached to long purple spring and hooked to the crossbar behind (find level that suits—increase or decrease resistance).
   Bend leg to a 60-degree angle with the foot soft.

> Inhale to prepare.
> Exhale to take the leg down, making an arch shape with the toe so that the leg moves from the hip only (don't increase the bend or straighten the knee).
> Inhale to take back to starting position.
> Repeat until hamstrings feel warmed.
> Straighten the leg up to the ceiling and gently stretch the hamstrings for about 5 breaths.

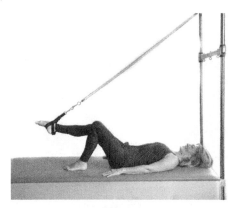

Figure 160

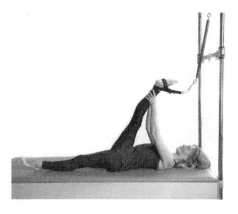

Figure 161

- Make sure the leg moves from the hip only keeping the 60-degree shape
- Support the head with a cushion
- Try to gradually increase the stretch at the end—don't force into a maximum stretch initially.

60. Eyelash exercise

Benefits: *strengthens the hamstrings and glutei*
Muscle focus: *glutei, hamstrings, pelvic stabilisers*

Lie face down with legs straight, bend your elbows, and rest your forehead on your hands. Slightly bend one knee so that the foot flexes and the toenail only is touching the floor.

Inhale to prepare.
Exhale as you draw in gently with the deep abdominal muscles, squeeze your buttocks as above, and try to just straighten the bent knee without putting any pressure on the toenail.

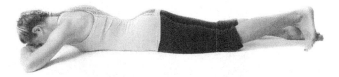

Figure 162

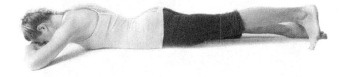

Figure 163

- Try to hold the spine in neutral in this position—don't let the back arch
- Feel the top of the back of the leg (hamstrings) connecting with the lower part of your buttock
- Imagine the toenail is an eyelash and you mustn't squash it as you straighten the leg.

61. Standing hip strengthener on combo chair

Benefits: *strengthens the hip flexors, quadriceps, and hamstrings while stabilising the pelvis; recruiting the gluteus medius helps to improve balance*
Muscle focus: *hip flexors, hamstrings, quadriceps, pelvic stabilisers*

2 x black springs (lowest hook).
  Stand facing the stool with one foot on the pedal. Standing foot parallel.
  Arms out to side or holding the handles or push through bar of trapeze.

  Exhale to push down pedal (stop just before hitting the floor); maintain an
  upright posture.
  Inhale to return to the starting position.

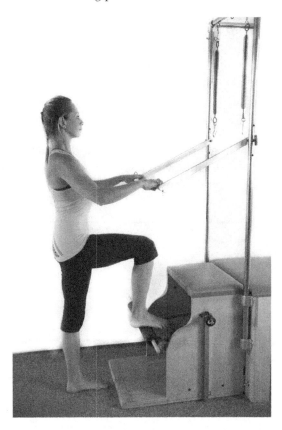

Figure 164

- Maintain pelvic stabilisation throughout
- Do not sink into standing hip
- Keep upright posture
- Working leg should move independently from the hip joint.

CHAPTER TWELVE

Spinal extension

62. Swimming prep

Benefits: *strengthens the erector spinae, middle and lower trapezius, glutei and hamstrings while stabilising the pelvis*
Muscle focus: *spinal extensors, hip extensors, scapula stabilisers, pelvic stabilisers*

Lie face down with your legs straight and your arms stretched up by your ears. Place a soft book or towel under your forehead.

Inhale to prepare, exhale as you draw in gently with the deep abdominal muscles, and lift your right arm and left leg slightly off the floor.
Inhale to return to the starting position.
Exhale and repeat on other side.

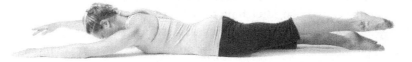

Figure 165

- Place a pillow under your tummy if you feel discomfort in your lower back
- Don't expect to lift the arm or leg very high off the ground
- Try to keep the shoulders drawn down your back
- Try not to lift the hip of the working leg.

63. Dart

Benefits: *strengthens the upper back extensors and lengthens the neck extensors while stabilising the shoulder and pelvic girdle*
Muscle focus: *scapula stabilisers, spinal extensors, pelvic stabilisers*

Lie face down with your legs straight and hands palms down by your shoulders with elbows pointing up to the ceiling.
   Place a cushion or soft book under your forehead.

>   Inhale to prepare, exhale as you draw in with the deep abdominal muscles, lengthen the tailbone towards your feet, and push the elbows down to the floor. Once you feel the shoulder blades pulling down lift the upper back and head keeping the chin down towards your chest.
>   Inhale to return to the starting position.

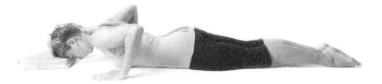

Figure 166

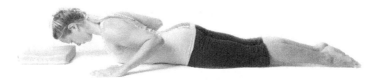

Figure 167

- Place a pillow under your tummy if you feel discomfort in your lower back, or under your hips if they are initially too tight to stretch fully
- Don't lift the shoulders and head too far off the floor
- Keep the chin down, stretching the back of the neck
- The neck should stay long at the back, in line with your spine: imagine that you have a glass of water balancing on your neck that you don't want to spill.

64. Diamond press

Benefits: *strengthens the upper back extensors while stabilising the shoulder and pelvic girdle*
Muscle focus: *spinal extensors, scapula stabilisers, pelvic stabilisers*

Lie face down with your legs straight; your arms should be bent and your hands in a diamond shape under your forehead with the thumb and forefingers touching.

Inhale to prepare, exhale as you draw in with the deep abdominal muscles and lengthen the tailbone towards the feet. Press gently down onto your forearms, lifting the upper back and head off the floor.
Inhale and return to the starting position.

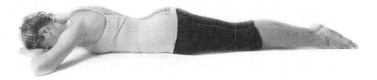

Figure 168

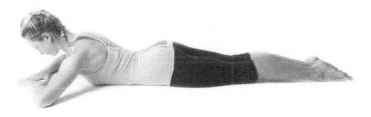

Figure 169

- Place a pillow under your tummy if you feel discomfort in your lower back or under your hips if they are initially too tight to stretch fully
- Don't lift the shoulders and head too far off the floor
- Initially lift the chin very slightly (imagine you are pushing a marble away with your nose), then keep the neck in line with the spine (keep chin down)
- Draw the shoulder blades down as you press into the floor with the forearms
- Feel your upper torso lifting off the floor while the rest of the body remains still.

65. Arrow

Benefits: *strengthens the upper back extensors while stabilising the shoulder and pelvic girdle*
Muscle focus: *spinal extensors, scapula stabilisers, arm extensors, pelvic stabilisers*

Lie face down with your legs straight; your arms should be by your side with palms facing up.
Place a cushion or soft book under your forehead.

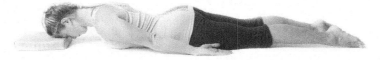

Figure 170

Inhale to prepare, exhale as you draw in with the deep abdominal muscles and lengthen the tailbone towards the feet. Float your arms up to the ceiling, then draw the shoulder blades down your back and lift the upper back and head.

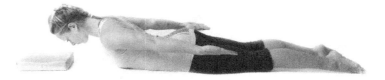

Figure 171

Inhale and return to the starting position.

- Place a pillow under your tummy if you feel discomfort in your lower back
- Don't lift the shoulders and head too far off the floor
- Keep the neck in line with the spine (keep chin down)
- Draw the shoulder blades down as you lift the upper back
- Keep the arms long but soft (don't lock the elbows).

66. Cobra

Benefits: *strengthens the upper back extensors while stabilising the shoulder and pelvic girdle*
Muscle focus: *spinal extensors, scapula stabilisers, elbow flexors, pelvic stabilisers*

Lie face down with your legs straight; your arms should be bent with elbows just above your shoulders and palms in line with elbows and facing inwards or down towards the floor.
    Place a cushion or soft book under your forehead.

Inhale to prepare, exhale as you draw in with the deep abdominal muscles and lengthen the tailbone towards the feet; draw the shoulder blades down your back and lift the upper back and head, pushing into your forearms.
Hold that position while you inhale again.
As you exhale lift the hands off the floor, keeping the elbows in contact with the floor.
Inhale to lower forearms and then lift again as you exhale.
Repeat the arm lift 3 times then lower back to start position.

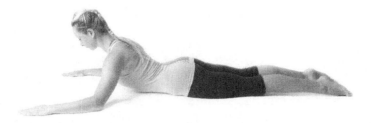

Figure 172

- Keep the shoulders drawing down throughout.
- Keep the abdominals and hip extensors engaged.
- Keep the head in line with spine.

67. Swan prep on reformer

Benefits: strengthens the upper back extensors using light resistance
Muscle focus: spinal extensors, scapula stabilisers, shoulder flexors, elbow extensors, elbow flexors, pelvic stabilisers

Springs: medium.
Place the long box on the reformer carriage.

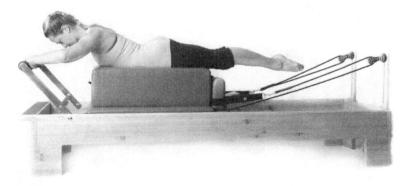

Figure 173

Lie on the carriage face down with edge of box about chest level and your hands on the foot bar with elbows bent outward and fingers pointing inwards slightly.

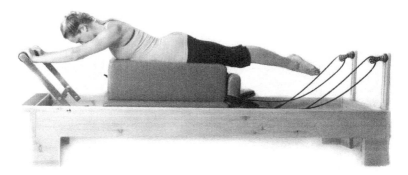

Figure 174

Inhale to prepare.

Exhale as you draw in with the deep abdominal muscles and lengthen the tailbone towards the feet. Feel the back of the legs engage and draw the shoulder blades down your back as you push away from the bar, lengthening the arms and rotating the hands to point straight ahead.

Inhale, then exhale to lift into back extension, keeping the shoulders down. Inhale and return to flat still with arms long.

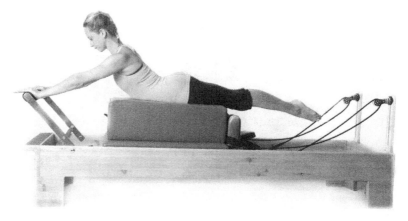

Figure 175

Exhale and open the elbows as they bend and return the carriage back to the starting position.

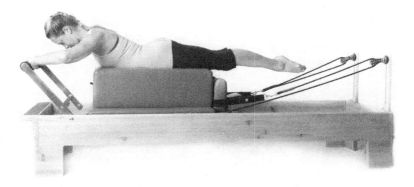

Figure 176

- Keep the shoulders drawing down throughout
- Keep the abdominals and hip extensors engaged
- Keep the fingers long and swivel the hands rather than gripping the bar
- Keep the head in line with spine.

68. Swan on combo chair

Benefits: strengthens the back extensors, mobilises the spine
Muscle focus: spinal extensors, scapular stabilisers, pelvic stabilisers

Lie prone over chair with legs straight
(resting on trapeze or reformer box stand)

Springs: low/medium.
Align shoulders directly over hands with arms straight.
  Inhale and allow pedals to lift body.

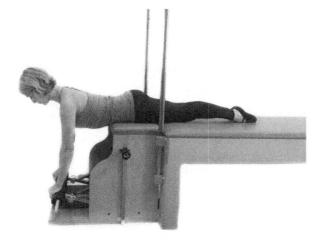

Figure 177

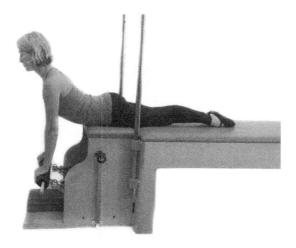

Figure 178

- Keep arms straight
- Keep head in line with spine
- Keep scapulae stabilised
- Engage abdominals and hip extensors to support lumbar spine
- Extend through whole of spine
- Lighten the springs to challenge the back extensors.

Four point kneeling

69. Superman

Benefits: *strengthens the deep posterior spinal stabilisers, shoulder girdle, glutei, and hamstrings while stabilising the pelvis*
Muscle focus: *scapula stabilisers, spinal extensors, hip extensors, shoulder flexors, pelvic stabilisers*

Start on all fours; your hips should be over the knees and your shoulders over your hands.

Inhale to prepare, exhale as you draw in with the deep abdominal muscles,
and lift right arm and left leg slightly off the floor.
Inhale to return to the starting position.
Exhale and repeat on the other side.

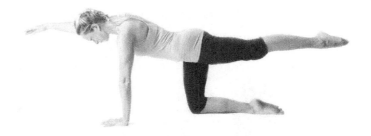

Figure 179

- Draw the abdominals up towards the spine at the start of the exercise to sta-bilise the torso
- Don't take the leg or arm too high, your lower back should not arch
- Be aware that the limbs which aren't moving are working to stabilise, so feel those connections with serratus (under arm) and opposite inner thigh muscles
- Keep the back of the neck long (don't lift the chin)
- The abdominals, back muscles and buttocks should work in unison to hold the torso still whilst lifting the limbs.

70. Superman on reformer

Benefits: strengthens the deep posterior spinal stabilisers, shoulder girdle, glutei, and ham-strings while stabilising the pelvis
Muscle focus: scapula stabilisers, spinal extensors, hip extensors, shoulder flexors, pelvic stabilisers

Springs: medium.
Start kneeling on the reformer with the hands on the shoulder rests, knees directly below hips, then place one foot behind on the foot bar so that the knee is slightly lifted off the carriage.

Inhale to prepare—make sure the shoulders are stabilised and the pelvis is level.
Exhale, draw the abdominals up towards the spine, and using the strength from the lifted leg push away from the bar keeping the pelvis level.

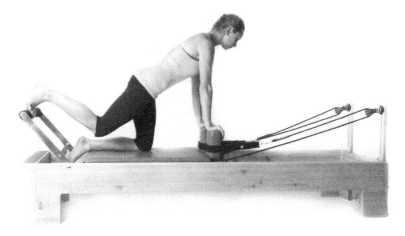

Figure 180

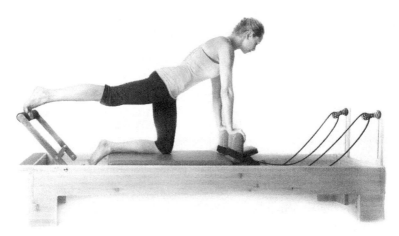

Figure 181

- Draw the abdominals up towards the spine at the start of the exercise to stabilise the torso
- Don't let your lower back arch as the leg extends
- Engage the gluteal muscles to keep the pelvis level
- Don't lead with the kneeling leg, keep the knee under the hip throughout
- Don't lock the elbows
- Keep the back of the neck long (don't lift the chin).

CHAPTER THIRTEEN

Spinal mobilisation

71. Thread the needle

Benefits: *stretches the middle back and shoulder girdle*

Start on all fours with your hips over the knees and shoulders over the hands.

Inhale, exhale as you draw in the deep abdominal muscles, and reach with one hand under the opposite arm and knee in the direction of the hip. Inhale as you bring the arm back and stretch it up to the ceiling.

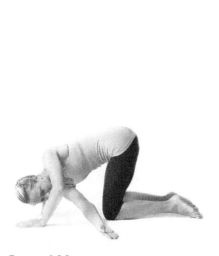

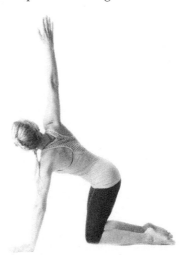

Figure 182

Figure 183

- Allow the shoulder of the moving arm to drop towards the floor
- Keep the neck relaxed following the direction of the moving arm
- Think of the arm threading through the hole of the needle and feel the stretch around the shoulder blades.

72. Lumbar circles

Benefits: *stretches the lumbar extensors and releases the sacro iliac joints*

Start lying semi supine. Lift one leg to table top then the other holding on to each knee.

Inhale to prepare.
Exhale to take both knees to your chest.
Exhale again and make little circles with your knees moving around the back of your pelvis in a circular movement.
Repeat circling the other way.

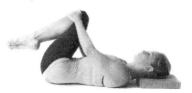

Figure 184

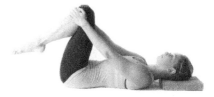

Figure 185

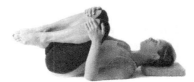

Figure 186

- Just breathe gently into the circles as you feel your lumbar spine and sacrum mobilising.

73. Small hip rolls

Benefits: *releases the sacro iliac joints and gently stretches the hip abductors*
Muscle focus: *hip abductors, pelvic stabilisers*

Start lying on your back with your legs bent over a gym ball and arms slightly out to side.

Inhale to prepare.
Exhale, draw in the abdominals, and roll over to one hip slightly lifting the other off the floor.

Inhale.

Exhale to activate the abdominals again and roll over the sacrum to the other hip.

Gently roll over the sacrum from one hip to the other keeping the control from the abdominal muscles.

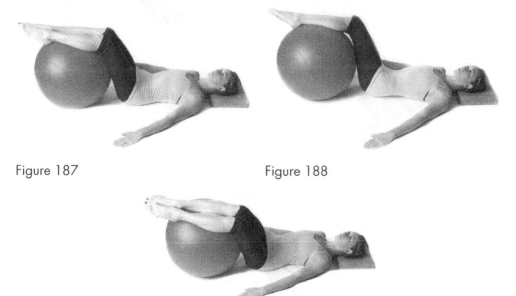

Figure 187   Figure 188

Figure 189

- Keep the knees in line with the hips throughout
- Move from the pelvis; don't lead with the legs.

74. Large hip rolls

Benefits: *stretches the hip abductors and spinal rotators*

Start lying on your back with your legs bent wider than hip width and arms out to the side.

Inhale to prepare.

Exhale, engage the abdominal muscles, and take both legs to one side letting the opposite hip lift, turning the head in the opposite direction.

Take a few breaths in that position, then when ready exhale to take the legs over to repeat on the other side.

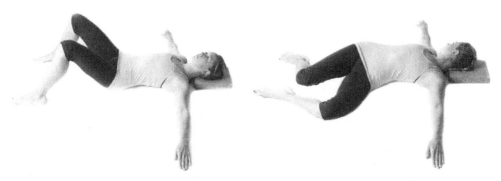

Figure 190   Figure 191

Make Make sure that the shoulders stay flat on the mat.

Progression

Once in the stretch lift the bottom foot and place on the top knee to increase
the stretch through the hip.
Place it back down before moving to the other side.

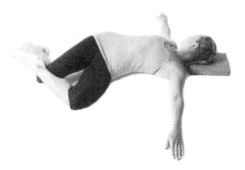

Figure 192

75. Cossack arms seated

Benefits: *mobilises the thoracic spinal rotators*
Muscle focus: *spinal rotators, scapular stabilisers, pelvic stabilisers*

Start seated on a chair or balance ball.
    Make sure knees are aligned and level with hips (place a book under feet if
necessary).
    Place one hand on top of other in front of chest with elbows held out to side and
thumbs touching the breastbone.

Inhale to prepare, exhale as you draw the abdominal muscles in, and rotate
the upper body to one side.

Inhale to return to centre.

Exhale and repeat to the other side.

- Keep the shoulders down and hands in middle of chest bone
- Try to keep the pelvis still and knees facing forward.

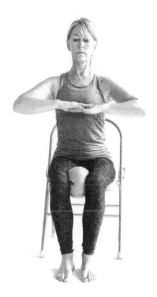

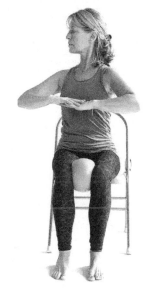

Figure 193   Figure 194

Modification for tight pecs or a kyphotic posture

Place a stick behind torso and wrap arms around it with palms facing forwards.

CHAPTER FOURTEEN

Knee and lower limb

76. Knee/ankle mobility exercise seated on reformer

Benefits: *mobilises the knee and ankle joints*
Muscle focus: *quadriceps, hamstrings, gastrocnemius, soleus, tibialis anterior*

No springs (remove the spring bar if able).

Sit on the reformer (sitting bones near the edge) facing the foot bar with your hands resting on the carriage.

Your feet should be flat on the floor and knees at right angles to the hips and in line with the toes (use blocks to raise feet if the reformer carriage is too high).

Inhale and sit tall.

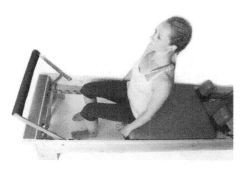

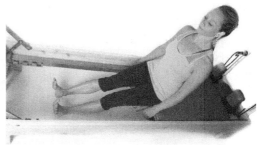

Figure 195   Figure 196

Exhale, draw the sitting bones together, engage the abdominals, and glide
backwards, straightening the legs and lifting the toes when necessary.
Inhale, lower the toes back down.
Exhale to bend the knees and draw the carriage back in tracking the knees
over the toes.

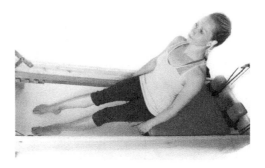

Figure 197

- Feel that you are lifting the knees up to the ceiling as they draw the carriage
  back in
- Keep sitting as upright as possible
- Don't use momentum or lead the movement with the torso
- Gradually increase the movement through the knees and ankles if possible.

77. Knee strengthening exercise seated on reformer

Benefits: *knee strengthening with resistance*
Muscle focus: *quadriceps, hamstrings, gastrocnemius, soleus*

1 yellow spring.
   Remove the shoulder pads and sit on the carriage facing the risers.
   Your feet should be flat on the floor and knees at right angles to the hips (use blocks
to raise feet if the reformer carriage is too high) with your toes in front of your knees
so that the legs are only slightly bent.

   Inhale and sit tall.
   Exhale, draw the sitting bones together, engage the abdominals, and glide
   forwards, tracking the knees over the toes.
   Inhale to return to the starting position.

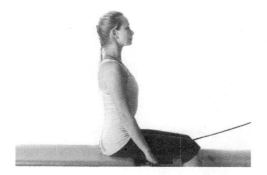

Figure 198

- Feel that you are lifting the knees up to the ceiling as they draw the carriage towards the feet
- Keep sitting as upright as possible
- Don't use momentum or lead the movement with the torso.

Modification

Repeat with one leg at a time, raising the other just off the floor.
Repeat again with the weaker knee.

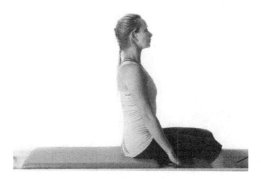

Figure 199

78. Standing knee stretch on reformer

Benefits: *quadriceps and hamstring strengthener with resistance and balance control*
Muscle focus: *quadriceps, hamstrings, pelvic stabilisers*

Springs: light.

Stand facing reformer on one straight parallel leg close to foot bar.
Place the ball of the other foot on edge of carriage.
Inhale to prepare.

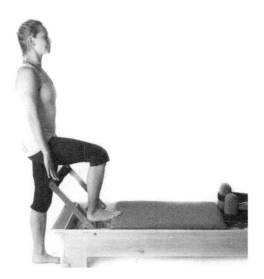

Figure 200

Exhale to push carriage away with the ball of the foot.

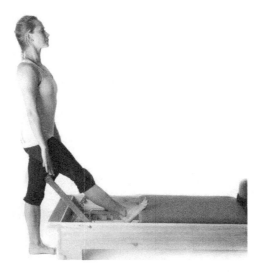

Figure 201

- Keep upright, do not tip body forward as knee extends
- Draw abdominals towards spine to maintain pelvic stabilisation.

79. Knee bend with TheraBand

Benefits: *quadriceps and hamstring strengthener with resistance*
Muscle focus: *quadriceps, hamstrings, pelvic stabilisers*

Lie on your back in neutral spine with your knees bent and feet hip width apart.

Lift one leg and place a TheraBand around the foot, holding each end in each hand with palms facing towards you and elbows bent by your side. Straighten the leg to a 45-degree angle.

Inhale to prepare.
Exhale as you engage the abdominals, draw down the shoulder blades, and bend the knee to 90 degrees, pushing the foot away against the resistance of the band.
Inhale and return the leg to the straight position.

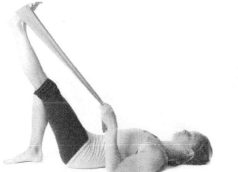

Figure 202

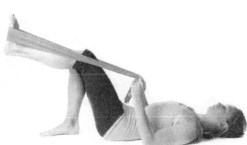

Figure 203

- Use the TheraBand to create resistance in the leg by bending from the knee only
- Don't move the leg from the hip or draw the thigh towards you as the knee bends
- Careful not to flex at the wrists.

80. Remedial knee exercise

Benefits: *knee strengthening and balancing of surrounding muscles; alignment of knee and hip during rotation*
Muscle focus: *quadriceps, hamstrings, gastrocnemius, soleus, deep hip rotators*

Lie on your back with knees bent, prop up your head and shoulders with cushions if needed, and place a couple of rolled-up cushions under one leg so that it is bent at a 60-degree angle and the back of the leg is supported.

Keep your breath controlled throughout.

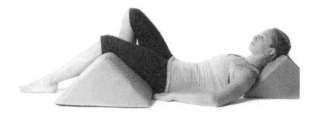

Figure 204

    1. Straighten the leg.

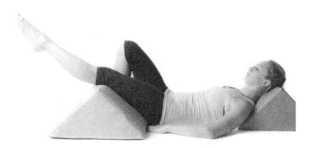

Figure 205

    2. Point the foot.

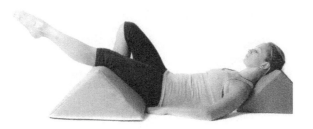

Figure 206

    3. Flex the foot (pull the toes back).

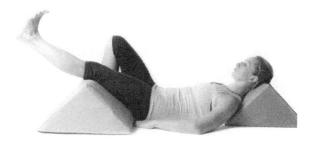

Figure 207

4. Externally rotate from the hip.

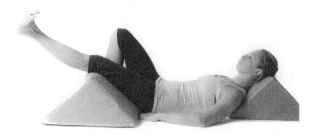

Figure 208

5. Rotate back to parallel.

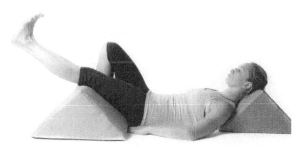

Figure 209

6. Relax the foot and bend the knee back to the starting position.

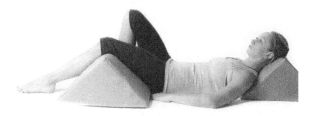

Figure 210

- Make sure the leg stays straight during hip rotation
- Rotate the leg from the hip only.

Progressions:

- On section 4 add: lift the leg towards the opposite shoulder (keeping externally rotated and foot flexed). Take the leg back to the support (keeping externally rotated and foot flexed) then continue with section 5
- Use a light ankle weight.

81. Knee strengthener with soft ball

Benefits: *strengthening of quadriceps medialis (last 25 degrees of extension); helps to stop hyper-extension of knees*
Muscle focus: *Vastus medialis*

Sit on the floor with legs outstretched and a soft Pilates ball under one knee.
Lean back onto hands just behind the hips, bend other leg if more comfortable.

Slowly lift the lower part of the leg to straight, gently pointing the foot without pushing down onto the ball.
Relax back down and repeat several times.
Repeat another set with the leg externally turned out from the hip.

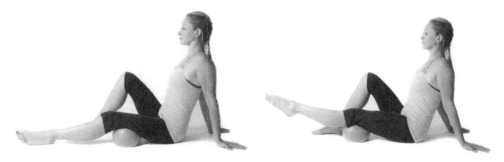

Figure 211   Figure 212

- Try to feel the muscles just above the kneecap engaging rather than the bulk of the quads
- Don't let the knee hyper-extend.

82. Leg work—wide position on reformer

Benefits: *helps to strengthen the muscles around the knee joint*
Muscle focus: *quadriceps (especially vastus medialis), hamstrings, pelvic stabilisers*

Start with balls of the feet on the bar in a wide V position (edge of bar), heels slightly lifted and externally rotated from the hip joints.

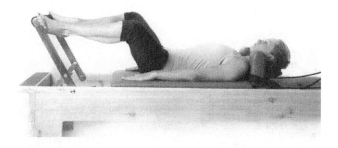

Figure 213

Inhale to prepare.
Exhale, and holding neutral push back to full extension keeping the heels
slightly lifted.
Inhale at top.
Exhale and bend the knees up to the ceiling, drawing the carriage back to
the starting position without moving the heels.

- Maintain neutral spine throughout
- Keep heels slightly raised and don't let them drop or lift higher so as to work
  through the knee and hip joints only
- Weight should stay evenly distributed across toe joints
- Don't externally over-rotate from the hips
- Maintain alignment of feet, knees, and hip joint.

83. Foot work with board on reformer

Benefits: knee and ankle strengthening and mobilising without weight bearing
Muscle focus: quadriceps, hamstrings, gastrocnemius, soleus, tibialis anterior

Springs: medium.

Lie supine with feet parallel on jump board.

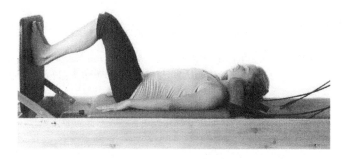

Figure 213a

Push back to full extension.

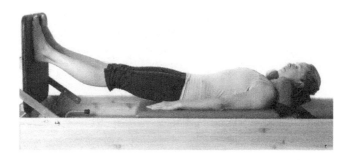

Figure 213b

Lift heels and transfer onto toe joints without pushing into board.
Lower heels.
Return to starting position lifting heels when necessary.

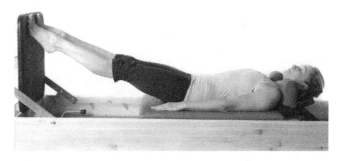

Figure 213c

- Maintain pelvic-lumbar stabilisation throughout
- Maintain alignment of hips, knees, and feet
- Weight should be evenly distributed across toe joints
- Straighten legs fully before lifting heels
- Use core strength to lift heels on rises rather than pushing into toe joints.

84. Ankle exercise on combo chair

Benefits: knee and ankle strengthening and mobilising without weight bearing
Muscle focus: gastrocnemius, soleus, tibialis anterior, flexor halluces longus, flexor digitorum longus

2 x black springs, lowest hook.

Stand facing the chair with one foot on the floor and the other on the pedal (toes).
Lean forward, knee touching front of stool with the back leg straight.

Plantar flex the foot to push the pedal down, flexing at the toe joints.
Dorsiflex the foot allowing the pedal to rise.

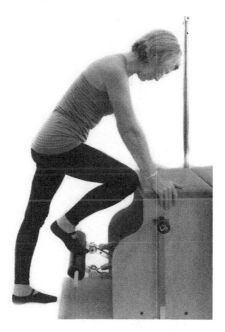

Figure 213d

- Make sure to distribute the weight between the big and second toe
- Lead with heel on dorsiflexion
- Keep the standing leg straight
- Keep both legs parallel.

CHAPTER FIFTEEN

Stretches

85. Quadriceps stretch

Benefits: stretches quadriceps

Stand holding on to a support

> Take hold of the foot of the leg to be stretched and bend behind towards your buttocks.
> Pull in the abdominals, push the tailbone down, and keep the knee facing downwards as much as possible.
> Breathe into the stretch and hold for at least 30 seconds.

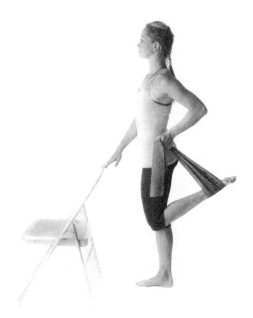

Figure 214

Modification

If you are unable to reach your foot behind, you can use a TheraBand wrapped around it to increase the range of movement.

86. Iliopsoas stretch standing

Benefits: *gently stretches iliopsoas*

Stand holding on to the back of a chair (or something else stable).
    Place the leg of the hip you want to stretch behind you with the foot on a low stool or seat of a sofa.

    Stand up as straight as possible and bend the standing leg.
    Move the stool as far away as needed to get a stretch through the front of the hip.

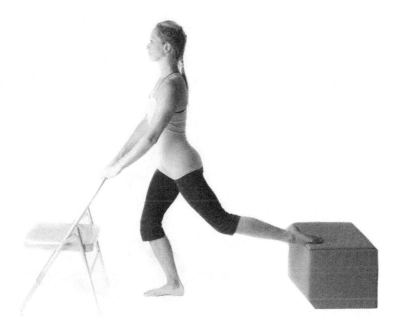

Figure 215

87. Iliopsoas stretch on a bed or treatment table (Thomas Test)

Benefits: *test for tightness and stretches iliopsoas*

Lie on the edge of a bed holding both knees to your chest with your back flat (use a headrest if needed).

> Let one leg go so that it hangs down off the edge of the bed pulling the other leg to your chest to maintain the flat back.
> You should feel the stretch through the front of the hip of the hanging leg.

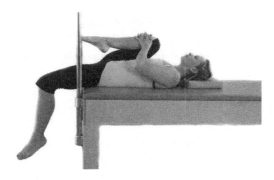

Figure 216

88. Iliopsoas and lumbar stretch on a soft ball

Benefits: *gently stretches iliopsoas*

Lie on your back in the rest position and place a soft Pilates ball under your sacrum.

Pull both knees to your chest and feel the stretch in the lumbar spine and breathe into this position.
Let one leg go and slide along the floor while keeping the other leg close to your chest.
Sink into the ball and feel the stretch deep into the hip of the outstretched leg as you breathe into this position.

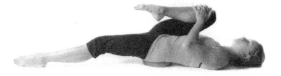

Figure 217

Change legs as necessary.

89. Iliopsoas stretch on reformer

Benefits: *stretches iliopsoas*

Light spring.

Stand close to the side of the frame holding on to the high foot bar or jump board with the other knee on the carriage and the foot touching the shoulder rest.

Inhale to prepare.
Exhale, engage the abdominals, and bend the standing knee while the other leg pushes the carriage back to obtain a stretch through the hip flexor.
Hold the stretch, breathe into it and try to increase the range of movement if possible.

- Keep as upright as possible and engage the abdominals to protect the lumbar spine
- Make sure the standing knee keeps above and in line with the toes.

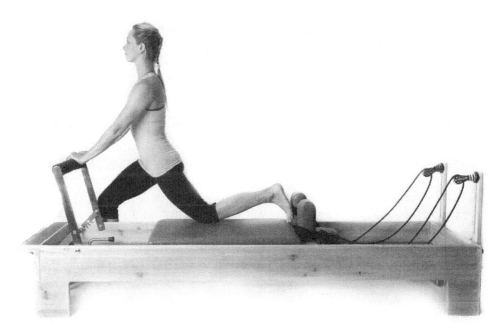

Figure 218

90. Buttock stretch

Benefits: *stretches the glutei*

Start semi supine.

   Place one bent leg in the air with a TheraBand wrapped around the thigh, bend the other and cross the foot over the lifted leg with the knee pointing outwards.

   Breathe in to prepare.
   Exhale and gently pull the band towards you so that the crossed leg is drawn towards the chest.
   Hold this position as you breathe until you feel the muscles relaxing.
   Repeat other side.

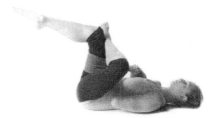

Figure 219

91. SI joint mobilisation on foam roller

Benefits: *mobilises SI joints and lumbar extensors*

Start lying semi supine.

> Lift the pelvis and place a foam roller under your sacrum level with the SI joints.
> Bend the knees towards your chest and hold the roller with your hands.
>
> Roll from side to side over your SI joints.
> Stay on one side and bring one knee at a time further towards your chest.
> Circle the knees around (close to your chest), massaging over the SI joint.
>
> • Keep the knees as close to your chest as possible throughout to keep the lumbar spine in flexion.

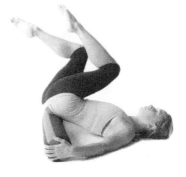

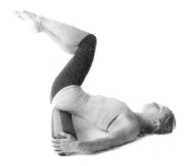

Figure 220   Figure 221

92. Pectoral stretch on roller

Benefits: *stretches and opens the chest*
Muscle focus: *pectoralis major, anterior deltoid*

Start lying lengthways on roller.

> Inhale to take arms to the ceiling.
> Exhale to take arms behind head and then bend into a right-angled position parallel to the floor with palms facing upwards.

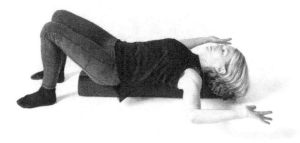

Figure 222

Alternative:

Take arms up to ceiling with palms facing inwards, then open to the side and breathe into the stretch.

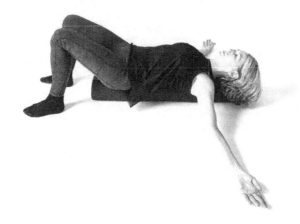

Figure 223

- Make sure neutral spine is held during this stretch; do not flare ribcage.

93. Around the world stretch

Benefits: *stretches and opens the chest*
Muscle focus: *pectoralis major, anterior deltoid*

Start lying on your side with legs bent to a comfortable position and head supported with a cushion. Arms outstretched level with the shoulders and palms together.

Inhale and take the top arm to the ceiling following the hand with your head. Exhale as you take it as far as you comfortably can over towards the floor the other side and breathe in that position.
Inhale to take back to the start position.

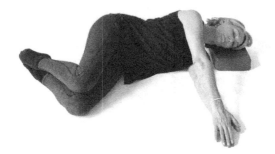

Figure 224

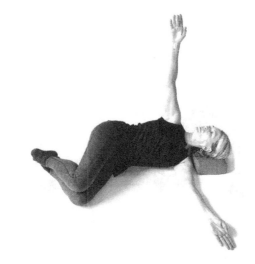

Figure 225

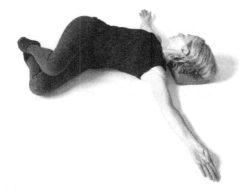

Figure 226

- Only go as far as you can without discomfort
- Use a pillow or support for the arm if the stretch position is causing discomfort
- Keep following the hand with the head.

94. Neck stretch

Benefits: *relieves tension in the neck and shoulders*
Muscle focus: *upper trapezius, levator scapulae*

Sit on a chair (or stand) with arms hanging down by your side.

Turn your head towards the direction of the tightness.
Incline your head so that the ear of the tight side lifts up to the ceiling and the chin points down to the armpit.
Feel the stretch coming from the top of the shoulder to the side of the neck.

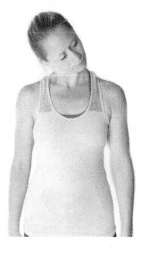

Figure 227

- Don't let the shoulders move, tilt, or rotate throughout
- The only movement is with the head.

95. Piriformis stretch

Benefits: *relieves tightness around the piriformis muscle which can be a cause of sciatica*

Start lying on your back, legs crossed at the knees in table top position.

Place the leg of the affected side on top.
Hold onto the ankles and pull the feet away from each other.
Breathe into stretch.

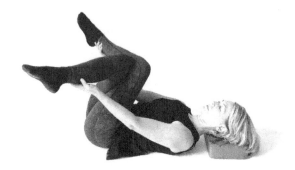

Figure 228

- Try to keep tailbone in contact with the floor
- Open the feet to the side (level with knees); don't pull downwards
- Use a band to wrap around one ankle if unable to reach with hand.

96. Lumbar stretch

Benefits: *lengthens the lumbar extensors*

Start lying semi supine. Lift one leg to table top then the other holding on to each knee.

Inhale to prepare.
Exhale to draw one knee to your chest.

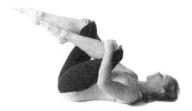

Figure 229

Inhale to return it to table top.
Exhale to draw the other knee to your chest.
Inhale to return.
Exhale to take both knees to your chest.

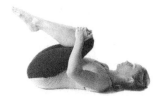

Figure 230

Breathe into this position feeling the stretch along the lumbar spine.

RESOURCES

Gunn, C. (2007). *Bones and Joints: A Guide for Students, Fifth Edition.* London: Churchill-Livingstone Elsevier.

Jarmey, C., & Sharkey, J. (2017). *The Concise Book of Muscle, Third Edition.* Chichester, UK: Lotus.

Sessa, S., & Pearce, K. (2020). *Pilates and Parkinson's* Aeon Books Ltd.

ACKNOWLEDGEMENTS

We had been planning to write this book for several years, but it took a pandemic and two national lockdowns to allow us both the time to do it!

We have spent many years running studios which specialise in rehabilitation through Pilates for clients and also more recently, teacher training courses which allow us to pass on our knowledge to other instructors.

We would like to thank Heidi Taylor of Studio 27 Photography for the beautiful photographs, Tom Ashfold for the wonderfully intricate anatomy drawings, and Eileen Hall for her full body drawings. Massive thanks also to Hannah Baker for being our Pilates model and Amy Oades for her time proofreading the text.

Lastly and most importantly the clients, physiotherapists, and Pilates instructors that we have worked with over the years, particularly Alan Herdman our "master trainer", and through whom we have gained the experience needed to write this book.

INDEX

abdominal exercise with gym ball or roller, 95–96. *See also* pelvic stabilisation exercises

achilles tendinopathy, 76–77. *See also* knee and lower leg

Achilles tendon (TA), 76

acute disc prolapse, 32. *See also* neck

adductor. *See also* pelvis and hip
  squeeze, 92
  strain, 60–61

adhesive capsulitis. *See* frozen shoulder

alignment, 6

ankle and foot, 69–70. *See also* knee and lower leg
  movements, 70

ankle exercise on combo chair, 184–185. *See also* knee and lower limb

ankle mobility exercise, 175–176. *See also* knee and lower limb

anterior cruciate ligaments (ACL), 69

anterior superior iliac spine (ASIS), 90

arm circles, 122–124. *See also* shoulder girdle

arm lifts, 112–113. *See also* shoulder girdle
  deltoid, 116–117
  standing, 113–114

around the world stretch, 193–195. *See also* stretches

arrow, 161–162. *See also* spinal extension

arthritic hip and joint replacement, 63. *See also* pelvis and hip

arthritis
  of glenohumeral joint, 49–50
  of knee and knee replacements, 74–76
  lumbar spine, 21

assisted bridge on trapeze, 103–104. *See also* pelvic stabilisation exercises

balance of body, 3

bone, 80

bone density and internal structure, 80

bone turnover, 80

breath, 4–5

breathing, 6. *See also* exercises; pelvic stabilisation exercises
  and deep core muscles, 89
  exercises, 89–90
  pilates rest position and basic, 91
  technique, 86
  technique using deep transversus abdominis muscles, 91

bridge, 102–103. *See also* pelvic stabilisation exercises

bug, 93–94. *See also* pelvic stabilisation exercises

bursae of the knee, 68
butterfly on soft ball, 106. *See also* pelvic
    stabilisation exercises
buttock stretch, 191. *See also* stretches

capsulitis, adhesive. *See* frozen shoulder
cartilage injuries of knee, 73–74
cat, the, 138–139. *See also* spinal flexion exercises
    on reformer, 139–140
cervical spine, 27. *See also* neck
    anatomical structures of, 27–28
    movements and muscles of, 29
cervical vertebrae, 27
cervicogenic headaches (CGH), 34–35.
        See also neck
chest lifts, 134–135. *See also* spinal flexion
        exercises
    oblique, 135–136
chin dips. *See also* shoulder girdle
    seated, 127
    on soft ball, 128
chondromalacia patella, 77. *See also* knee and
        lower leg
clam, 145–146. *See also* hip rehabilitation
cobra, 162–163. *See also* spinal extension
Contrology, 3
cossack arms, 121–122. *See also* shoulder girdle;
        spinal mobilisation
    seated, 172–173
curl down. *See also* spinal flexion exercises
    with TheraBand, 136
    on trapeze, 136–138

dart, 160. *See also* spinal extension
deep transversus abdominis muscles, 91
degenerative joint disease, 21–22, 29–30. *See also*
        lumbar spine; neck
deltoid arm lift, 116–117. *See also* shoulder
        girdle
diamond press, 160–161. *See also* spinal
        extension
disc degeneration. *See* spondylosis
disc prolapse, acute, 32. *See also* neck
dumb waiter, 107. *See also* shoulder girdle
    progressions, 108–109

exercises, 86, 89–90
    abdominal, 95–96
    breathing, 86, 89–90
    eyelash, 157

hamstring, 156–157
hip abductor, 147–149
knee/ankle mobility, 175–176
knee strengthening, 176–177
muscle focus, 86–88
pelvic stabilisation, 89
remedial knee, 179–181
serratus, 114–119
side lying hip, 146–147
spinal flexion, 131
eyelash exercise, 157. *See also* hip
    rehabilitation

facet joint syndrome, 20–21. *See also* lumbar
    spine
flat back, 11. *See also* posture
foot work, 183–184. *See also* knee and lower
    limb
four point kneeling, 166. *See also* spinal
    extension
    superman, 166–167
    superman on reformer, 167–168
frozen shoulder, 43–45. *See also* shoulder
functional scoliosis, 79

greater trochanteric pain syndrome (GTPS),
    54–55. *See also* pelvis and hip
groin strain, 60–61. *See also* pelvis and hip
gym ball
    abdominal exercise with, 95–96
    lumbar stretch seated with, 142–143
    seated with, 142–143

hamstring curls, 152–153. *See also* hip
    rehabilitation
    with extension, 153–154
    with extension, abduction, and adduction,
        154–155
hamstring exercise on trapeze, 156–157.
        See also hip rehabilitation
head rolls on soft ball, 129. *See also* shoulder
    girdle
hip, 52–53. *See also* pelvis and hip
    osteoarthritis of, 63–65
    replacement, 63
hip abductor exercise, 147–148. *See also*
        hip rehabilitation
    on trapeze, 148–149
hip and joint replacement, arthritic, 63.
        See also pelvis and hip

hip circles. *See also* hip rehabilitation
    on reformer, 150–151
    with TheraBand, 150
hip rehabilitation, 145
    clam, 145–146
    eyelash exercise, 157
    hamstring curls, 152–153
    hamstring curls with extension, 153–154
    hamstring curls with extension, abduction, and adduction, 154–155
    hamstring exercise on trapeze, 156–157
    hip abductor exercise, 147–148
    hip abductor exercise on trapeze, 148–149
    hip circles on reformer, 150–151
    hip circles with TheraBand, 150
    prone gluteal squeeze, 152
    side lying hip exercise, 146–147
    side lying leg work, 149–150
    standing hip strengthener, 157–158
hip rolls. *See also* spinal mobilisation
    large, 171–172
    small, 170–171
hyper-kyphosis, 10. *See also* posture
hyper-lordosis, 10. *See also* posture

iliopsoas, 58. *See also* pelvis and hip
    and lumbar stretch on soft ball, 190
    syndrome, 58–59
iliopsoas stretch. *See also* stretches
    on bed or table, 189
    on reformer, 190–191
    on soft ball, 190
    standing, 188–189
iliopsoas syndrome, 58–59. *See also* pelvis and hip
ilio-tibial band (ITB), 53, 54

joint disease, degenerative, 21–22, 29–30. *See also* lumbar spine; neck

knee, 67. *See also* knee and lower limb; pelvic stabilisation exercises
    bend with TheraBand, 178–179
    bursae of the, 68
    cartilage injuries of, 73–74
    drops, 94
    lifts, 94–95
    meniscal injuries of, 73–74
    mobility exercise, 175–176
    remedial knee exercise, 179–181

replacement, 74
    strengthener with soft ball, 182
    strengthening exercise, 176–177
knee and lower leg, 67
    achilles tendinopathy, 76–77
    anatomy, 67
    ankle and foot movements, 69–70
    arthritis and knee replacements, 74–76
    bursae of the knee, 68
    cartilage injuries, 73–74
    chondromalacia patella, 77
    conditions, 71
    knee joint, 67–69
    knee joint and menisci, 68
    knee joint movements, 69
    ligament injuries, 71–72
    Osgood Schlatter's disease, 77
    subtalar joint, 70
knee and lower limb, 175
    ankle exercise, 184–185
    foot work with board on reformer, 183–184
    knee/ankle mobility exercise, 175–176
    knee bend with TheraBand, 178–179
    knee strengthener with soft ball, 182
    knee strengthening exercise, 176–177
    leg work, 182–183
    remedial knee exercise, 179–181
    standing knee stretch, 177–178
knee joint, 67. *See also* knee and lower leg
    and menisci, 68
    movements, 69
kneeling, 114–116. *See also* pelvic stabilisation exercises
    four point, 166
    plank on reformer, 104

lateral collateral ligament (LCL), 68
leg slides, 93. *See also* pelvic stabilisation exercises
leg work, 96–102. *See also* knee and lower limb; pelvic stabilisation exercises
    wide position on reformer, 182–183
ligament injuries, 71–72. *See also* knee and lower leg
low back pain (LBP), 17–18
lower crossed syndrome, 81. *See also* postural dysfunction
lumbar circles, 170. *See also* spinal mobilisation
lumbar lordosis, 81. *See also* postural dysfunction

lumbar spine, 15
    anatomy of, 15
    arthritis of, 21
    conditions of, 17
    degenerative joint disease, 21–22
    facet joint syndrome, 20–21
    low back pain, 17–18
    lumbar vertebrae, 16
    movement, 16–17
    prolapsed intervertebral disc, 18–20
    spinal stenosis, 25–26
    spondylolysis and spondylolisthesis, 23–24
    vertebral column, 15
lumbar stretch, 196. *See also* spinal flexion
    exercises; stretches
    seated on reformer, 142
    seated with gym ball, 142–143
    on soft ball, 190
lumbar vertebrae, 16

medial collateral ligament (MCL), 69
meniscal injury, 73. *See also* knee and lower leg
    of knee, 73–74
mini curl up with push-through bar on trapeze,
    140–142. *See also* spinal flexion
    exercises
movements and muscles
    of cervical spine and head, 29
    of knee joint, 69
    pelvis and hip joints, 53
    of shoulder girdle and shoulder joint, 38
muscle
    balance, 6–9
    focus, 86–88
    of shoulder joint, 39
    that move and stabilise scapula, 39

National Institute for Health and Care
    Excellence (NICE), x
neck, 27. *See also* stretches
    acute disc prolapse, 32
    anatomical structures of cervical spine,
    27–28
    atlas, 28
    axis, 28
    cervical vertebrae, 27
    cervicogenic headaches, 34–35
    common conditions of, 29
    degenerative joint disease, 29–30

    movements and muscles of cervical spine
    and head, 29
    stretch, 195
    torticollis, 33–34
    whiplash, 30–32
neutral spine, 90. *See also* pelvic stabilisation
    exercises
non-specific low back pain (NSLBP), 17–18.
    See also lumbar spine

oblique chest lifts, 135–136
Osgood Schlatter's disease, 77. *See also* knee
    and lower leg
osteitis pubis, 61–62. *See also* pelvis and hip
osteoarthritis, 22. *See also* pelvis and hip
    of hip and hip replacement, 63–65
osteoporosis, 80. *See also* postural dysfunction

pars interarticularis (PI), 23
partial knee replacement (PKR), 75
patella, chondromalacia, 77. *See also* knee and
    lower leg
pectoral stretch on roller, 192–193. *See also*
    stretches
pelvic curls seated on reformer, 133–134.
    See also spinal flexion exercises
pelvic floor activation, 91–92. *See also* pelvic
    stabilisation exercises
pelvic girdle, 51–52
pelvic stabilisation exercises, 89. *See also*
    exercises
    abdominal exercise with gym ball or roller,
    95–96
    adductor squeeze, 92
    anterior tilt, 90
    assisted bridge on trapeze, 103–104
    breathing and deep core muscles, 89
    breathing exercises, 89–90
    breathing technique using deep transversus
    abdominis muscles, 91
    bridge, 102–103
    bug, 93–94
    butterfly on soft ball, 106
    knee drops, 94
    knee lifts, 94–95
    kneeling plank on reformer, 104
    leg slides, 93
    leg work, 96–102
    neutral, 90

neutral spine, 90
pelvic floor activation, 91–92
pilates rest position and basic breathing, 91
posterior tilt, 90
prancers, 102
tippy toes on soft ball, 105–106
pelvic tilts, 131–132. *See also* spinal flexion
    exercises
    larger, 132–133
    small, 132
    on soft pilates ball, 132
pelvis and hip, 51
    anatomy of, 51
    arthritic hip and joint replacement, 63
    conditions, 54
    greater trochanteric pain syndrome, 54–55
    groin strain, 60–61
    hip, 52–53
    hip replacement, 63
    iliopsoas syndrome, 58–59
    joints, 52–53
    movement of pelvis and hip joints, 53
    osteitis pubis, 61–62
    osteoarthritis of hip and hip replacement,
        63–65
    pelvic girdle, 51–52
    piriformis syndrome, 57–58
    pubic symphysis pain, 61
    sacroiliac dysfunction, 56–57
    sacroiliac joint pain, 56
Pilates. *See also* pelvic stabilisation exercises
    fundamentals, 6
    rehabilitation through, ix
    rest position and basic breathing, 91
    six principles of, 4
pilates ball, small pelvic tilts on soft, 132
Pilates, J., 3
Pilates method basics, 3. *See also* Pilates
    alignment, 6
    back of skeleton, 5
    balance of body, 3
    breath, 4–5
    breathing, 6
    centre, 6
    centring, 6
    concentration, 5
    control, 6
    flat back, 11
    flow, 6

front of skeleton, 4
    hyper-kyphosis, 10
    hyper-lordosis, 10
    muscle balance, 6–9
    muscles, 7–8
    posture, 9–11
    precision, 6
    sway back, 11
piriformis stretch, 195–196. *See also* stretches
piriformis syndrome, 57–58. *See also* pelvis
    and hip
poor seated posture, 79
posterior cruciate ligaments (PCL), 69
posterior tilt, 90
postural dysfunction, 79
    bone density and internal structure, 80
    functional scoliosis, 79
    lower crossed syndrome, 81
    lumbar lordosis and thoracic kyphosis, 81
    osteoporosis, 80
    poor seated posture, 79
    structural scoliosis, 79
    upper crossed syndrome, 82
posture, 9. *See also* Pilates method basics
    flat back, 11
    hyper-kyphosis, 10
    hyper-lordosis, 10
    sway back, 11
prancers, 102. *See also* pelvic stabilisation
    exercises
precision, 6
prolapsed intervertebral disc (PID), 17–20, 29.
    See also lumbar spine
prone gluteal squeeze, 152. *See also* hip
    rehabilitation
pubic symphysis pain, 61. *See also* pelvis and
    hip

quadriceps stretch, 187–188. *See also* stretches

range of movement (ROM), 16
reformer
    cat on, 139–140
    foot work with board on, 183–184
    hip circles on, 150–151
    iliopsoas stretch on, 190–191
    knee/ankle mobility exercise seated on,
        175–176
    kneeling plank on, 104

knee strengthening exercise seated on,
      176–177
leg work, 96–102
leg work wide position on, 182–183
lumbar stretch seated on, 142
pelvic curls seated on, 133–134
prep on, 163–165
seated plough on reformer box, 111–112
side lying leg work on, 149–150
standing knee stretch on, 177–178
superman on, 167–168
swan prep on, 163–165
Universal Reformer machine, 3
rehabilitation through Pilates, ix
remedial knee exercise, 179–181. *See also* knee
      and lower limb
roller, abdominal exercise with, 95–96.
            See also pelvic stabilisation exercises
rotator cuff disorders, 40–43. *See also* shoulder

sacroiliac (SI), 53. *See also* pelvis and hip;
            stretches
      dysfunction, 56–57
      joint mobilisation on foam roller, 192
      joint pain, 56
scapula dyskinesis, 48
scapulohumeral rhythm, 39–40.
            See also shoulder
scapulothoracic joint, 37
scoliosis, 79. *See also* postural dysfunction
seated on reformer, 142
seated plough, 109–111. *See also* shoulder girdle
      on reformer box, 111–112
serratus. *See also* shoulder girdle
      cushion squeeze, 114
      exercise with springs, 118–119
      exercise with TheraBand, 114–118
shoulder, 37
      anatomy, 37–38
      arthritis of glenohumeral joint, 49–50
      common conditions, 40
      dislocation, 45
      frozen, 43–45
      impingement, 41
      instability, 45–47
      joint, 38
      joint release, 130
      mobilisation with push through bar on
            trapeze, 126–127
      mobilisation with TheraBand, 124–125

movements of, 38
muscles of, 39
rehab, 120–121
rotator cuff disorders, 40–43
scapula dyskinesis, 48–49
scapula muscles, 39
scapulohumeral rhythm, 39–40
scapulothoracic joint, 37
winging scapula, 47
shoulder girdle, 107. *See also* serratus;
            shoulder
      arm circles, 122–124
      arm lifts, 112–113
      chin dips, 127–128
      cossack arms, 121–122
      deltoid arm lift, 116–117
      dumb waiter, 107–109
      head rolls on soft ball, 129
      seated plough, 109–111
      seated plough on reformer box, 111–112
      and shoulder joint, 38
      shoulder joint release, 130
      standing arm lift, 113–114
side lying hip exercise, 146–147. *See also* hip
            rehabilitation
side lying leg work on reformer, 149–150.
            See also hip rehabilitation
skeleton, 4–5
small hip rolls, 170–171. *See also* spinal
            mobilisation
soft ball. *See also* shoulder girdle
      butterfly on, 106
      chin dips on soft ball, 128
      head rolls on, 129
      iliopsoas and lumbar stretch on, 190
      knee strengthener with soft ball, 182
      tippy toes on, 105–106
spinal extension, 159
      arrow, 161–162
      cobra, 162–163
      dart, 160
      diamond press, 160–161
      four point kneeling, 166
      superman, 166–167
      superman on reformer, 167–168
      swan on combo chair, 165–166
      swan prep on reformer, 163–165
      swimming prep, 159
spinal flexion exercises, 131. *See also* exercises
      cat, the, 138–140

chest lifts, 134–135
curl down on trapeze, 136–138
curl down with TheraBand, 136
larger pelvic tilts, 132–133
lumbar stretch seated on reformer, 142
lumbar stretch seated with gym ball, 142–143
mini curl up with push-through bar on trapeze, 140–142
oblique chest lifts, 135–136
pelvic curls seated on reformer, 133–134
pelvic tilts, 131–132
small pelvic tilts on soft pilates ball, 132
spinal mobilisation, 169
cossack arms seated, 172–173
large hip rolls, 171–172
lumbar circles, 170
small hip rolls, 170–171
thread the needle, 169–170
spinal stenosis, 25–26. *See also* lumbar spine
spondylolisthesis, 23–24. *See also* lumbar spine
spondylolysis, 23–24. *See also* lumbar spine
spondylosis, 22, 30
standing arm lift, 113–114
standing hip strengthener on combo chair, 157–158. *See also* hip rehabilitation
standing knee stretch, 177–178. *See also* knee and lower limb
sternocleidomastoid (SCM), 29
stretches, 187
around the world, 193–195
buttock stretch, 191
iliopsoas and lumbar, 190
iliopsoas stretch on bed or table, 189
iliopsoas stretch on reformer, 190–191
iliopsoas stretch standing, 188–189
lumbar, 196
neck, 195
pectoral stretch on roller, 192–193
piriformis, 195–196
quadriceps, 187–188
SI joint mobilisation on foam roller, 192
around the world, 193–195
structural scoliosis, 79
subtalar joint, 70
superman, 166–167. *See also* four point kneeling on reformer, 167–168
supine, 117–118
swan. *See also* spinal extension
on combo chair, 165–166
prep on reformer, 163–165

sway back, 11. *See also* posture
swimming prep, 159. *See also* spinal extension

tendinopathy, achilles, 76–77. *See also* knee and lower leg
tension-type headaches (TTH), 35
tensor facia lata (TFL), 53
TheraBand
curl down with, 136
hip circles with, 150
knee bend with TheraBand, 178–179
serratus exercise with, 114–118
shoulder mobilisation with, 124–125
Thomas test, 189. *See also* stretches
abdominal exercise with gym ball or roller, 95–96
ankle exercise on combo chair, 184–185
breathing exercises, 89–90
thoracic kyphosis, 81. *See also* postural dysfunction
thread the needle, 169–170. *See also* spinal mobilisation
tippy toes on soft ball, 105–106. *See also* pelvic stabilisation exercises
torticollis, 33–34. *See also* neck
total knee replacement (TKR), 75
trapeze
assisted bridge on, 103–104
curl down on, 136–138
hamstring exercise on, 156–157
hip abductor exercise on, 148–149
mini curl up with push-through bar on, 140–142
serratus exercise with springs, 118–119
shoulder mobilisation with push through bar on, 126–127

Universal Reformer machine, 3
upper crossed syndrome, 82. *See also* postural dysfunction

vertebral column, 15

whiplash, 30–32. *See also* neck
winging
scapula, 47
of scapula and scapula dyskinesis, 47–49

Made in United States
North Haven, CT
21 September 2024

57710536R00122